MEDICINE AND HEALING
IN THE PREMODERN WEST

THE **BROADVIEW**
SOURCES SERIES

Medicine and Healing in the Premodern West

A HISTORY IN DOCUMENTS

edited by WINSTON BLACK

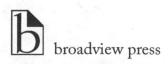
broadview press

BROADVIEW PRESS – www.broadviewpress.com
Peterborough, Ontario, Canada

Founded in 1985, Broadview Press remains a wholly independent publishing house. Broadview's focus is on academic publishing; our titles are accessible to university and college students as well as scholars and general readers. With over 600 titles in print, Broadview has become a leading international publisher in the humanities, with world-wide distribution. Broadview is committed to environmentally responsible publishing and fair business practices.

Library and Archives Canada Cataloguing in Publication

Title: Medicine and healing in the premodern West : a history in documents / edited by Winston Black.
Names: Black, Winston E., 1977– editor.
Series: Broadview sources series.
Description: Series statement: The Broadview sources series | Includes bibliographical references.
Identifiers: Canadiana (print) 20190159081 | Canadiana (ebook) 20190159111 | ISBN 9781554813902 (softcover) | ISBN 9781770487192 (PDF) | ISBN 9781460406755 (HTML)
Subjects: LCSH: Medicine—History—Sources. | LCSH: Healing—History—Sources.
Classification: LCC R131 .M43 2019 | DDC 610.9—dc23

Broadview Press handles its own distribution in North America:
PO Box 1243, Peterborough, Ontario K9J 7H5, Canada
555 Riverwalk Parkway, Tonawanda, NY 14150, USA
Tel: (705) 743-8990; Fax: (705) 743-8353
email: customerservice@broadviewpress.com

Distribution is handled by Eurospan Group in the UK, Europe, Central Asia, Middle East, Africa, India, Southeast Asia, Central America, South America, and the Caribbean. Distribution is handled by Footprint Books in Australia and New Zealand.

Canada Broadview Press acknowledges the financial support of the Government of Canada for our publishing activities.

Copy-edited by Juliet Sutcliffe
Book design by Em Dash Design

PRINTED IN CANADA

CONTENTS

PREFACE AND ACKNOWLEDGEMENTS

The history of medicine has grown rapidly as a field of research and study in the last decade or so. Schools across the United States, Canada, and the United Kingdom have increased the number of classes and programs in this field, at a time when other areas of the humanities are being diminished or cut. I have had the pleasure of being a part of this growth in medical history, teaching several college seminars on the history of medicine over the last decade. In these courses I explore the shifting interpretations of sickness and healing during Antiquity and the Middle Ages with my students. I also teach introductory surveys of Western Civilization, where I introduce students to the importance of Hippocrates and humoral theory in the Western tradition, if only in a single class session. This volume found its genesis between those two poles, as I identified specific sources or types of documents that I wanted to share with students in both the surveys and the seminars, as well as with teachers or scholars looking for an introduction to ancient and medieval medicine. I am grateful to the administrations and history departments at Shippensburg University, Binghamton University, the University of Tennessee, and Clark University for encouraging me to teach courses on the history of science, medicine, and disease.

This book owes much to the organizers (Professor Monica Green and Professor Rachel Scott, both then of Arizona State University) and participants of the 2012 National Endowment for the Humanities Summer Seminar "Health and Disease in the Middle Ages," held in London at the Wellcome Library for the History of Medicine. Monica Green has become a dear friend and mentor since then, offering constant support in my career and research as a historian of medicine. Among the 2012 NEH participants, Jennifer Edwards, Nahyan Fancy, and Sara Ritchey helped most with this project by sharing texts and ideas. Many other historians of medicine and medieval culture also deserve mention here, who each helped in his or her own way: Nicole Archambeau, Gerrit Bos, Carmen Caballero Navas, Ann Carmichael, Luke Demaitre, Mary Dzon, Nicholas Everett, Lori Jones, John Riddle, Tess Tavormina, Anne Van Arsdall, Nükhet Varlık, and Faith Wallis.

I would like to thank the librarians and staff at the Assumption College D'Alzon Library, Clark University Goddard Library, Brown University John D. Rockefeller, Jr., Library, the Wellcome Library in London, and the Worcester Public Library, for their assistance in my research on this collection. Members of the online scholarly group MEDMED (the medieval medicine email listserv) and the Facebook groups for the Society for the Social History of Medicine and Teaching the Middle Ages also helped shape my ideas about this volume. Some of the ideas presented here also found genesis in the Medical Paleography research group, an international team of scholars of medieval medicine and medieval manuscripts and paleography, founded and directed by Monica Green. I am also grateful to Brett McLenithan, Stephen Latta, Tara Lowes, Joe Davies, Juliet Sutcliffe, and Merilee Atos of Broadview Press, along with the editorial board at Broadview and the anonymous reviewers, for helping to make this book a reality.

Finally, I dedicate this book to my wonderful boys, Gabriel and Eliot, who have grown so fast while I've written it, and to my wife Dr. Emily Reiner, also a medievalist and a professional editor, who has balanced tough criticism with loving support during this project.

East Pennant, Nova Scotia

INTRODUCTION

Everybody gets sick or hurt at some time in his or her life. This is as true now as it was one thousand or ten thousand years ago. Archaeological and documentary evidence suggests that every human culture has practiced some form of medicine to heal diseases, treat wounds, prolong life, or at least relieve suffering. The history of medicine is a reflection of all humanity at the same time as it reveals differences between cultures. The documents in this collection belong to the history of medicine in the broadest sense, as they record not only learned explanations of disease and the nature of the human body but also methods of healing which are no longer considered part of "medicine." These include prayers, pilgrimage, magical spells, and talismans, all of which were used together with the more traditional, "natural" methods of herbal remedies, dietary management, and surgery.

Despite the central role of medicine in all of human history, much of the medical practice in the past is now dismissed simply as wrong according to the standards of modern science. In the last century, we have grown accustomed to rapid advances in medicine, brought about by discoveries or inventions which seem to transform medical theory and practice almost overnight. These include the invention or discovery of vaccines, anesthesia, germ theory, antibiotics, contraceptives, and the science of genetics, all of which have vastly improved the quality and length of human life. Such rapid changes in medicine, and their undeniable successes in healing, have made it easy to reject and forget the medical systems of the past. It can be difficult for modern audiences to appreciate the significance of medical systems which dominated healing within a culture, without significant change, for centuries or even millennia. By our modern standard of constant progress, their failure to change much over time implies a similar failure to heal. Yet several influential medical systems were first developed at least 2,000 years ago and survived, without significant changes, for many centuries. These include traditional Chinese medicine (TCM), Indian Ayurvedic medicine, and the premodern Western medicine based on the teachings of **Hippocrates** and **Galen**. The first two medical systems, TCM and Ayurveda, are still practiced by millions of people around the world, often as "complementary" or "alternative" medicines together with modern biomedicine, pharmaceuticals, and medical technology.

We do a great disservice to our understanding of the human condition and of attempts to relieve human suffering if we simply dismiss all early or traditional medicine out of hand. Studying the healers and healing traditions of past cultures provides us with a window onto their understanding of the human body, of gender, of why and how people suffer, and of people's ability

Hippocrates: Hippocrates of Kos (ca. 460–ca. 370 BCE) was a Greek physician who practiced and taught medicine in Athens during the peak of classical Greece. A contemporary of Pericles and Socrates, Hippocrates is frequently considered the "father" of Western medicine for establishing a school of medical thought based on clinical observation and natural explanations for disease. Approximately 60 medical texts are attributed to his authorship although it is unclear if he actually wrote any of them.

Galen: Claudius Galenus of Pergamon (ca. 130–ca. 210 CE) is generally considered the greatest physician of Western antiquity after Hippocrates. A Greek physician born in the Roman Empire, Galen practiced medicine in Rome itself, eventually serving as imperial physician to Marcus Aurelius. Galen saw himself as the direct heir of Hippocrates and wrote hundreds of medical and philosophical texts explaining Hippocratic texts and elaborating the humoral theory attributed to Hippocrates.

I

to control and change their world. Every form of medicine, including those that we now consider right, is a product of a specific historical period and culture, and it benefits all historians (and not just historians of medicine in particular) to understand the contexts that created and promoted different forms of healing. The study of past medical cultures also shows us the roots of our current medical systems. Modern Western medicine did not appear out of nowhere in the last two centuries, but is a direct heir of several overlapping ancient and medieval medical traditions.

This book focuses on medicine in the premodern West, a term which includes the cultures of the Mediterranean basin, Near East, and Europe from the oldest medical writings in Ancient Egypt to the end of the Middle Ages (ca. 2000 BCE–ca. 1500 CE). While many historians have rightly criticized this and other definitions of "the West," it is an apt category when studying the history of medicine, because premodern medicine in this area of the world, despite the great variety of practices within that period, is clearly distinct from the medical cultures of Sub-Saharan Africa, South Asia, or East Asia. From the Atlantic Ocean to the Indian subcontinent, from Iceland to the Sahara Desert, polytheists, philosophers, Christians, Jews, and Muslims embraced similar and often overlapping medical theories and practices. By the Middle Ages, all of these cultures shared the texts or at least the influence of the **humoral medicine** of Hippocrates and Galen, but their medical system is only the most famous example of the variegated western medical tradition.

This book also focuses on premodern Western medicine because its dominant medical tradition of Hippocratic-Galenic humoralism has been forgotten when compared to still vibrant medical systems like TCM and Ayurveda.[1] You can find clinics practicing the latter forms of medicine today in any major city, but you will never find a "Hippocratic" medical clinic, even though all three traditions share a focus on balancing the humors or elements of the body to bring it back into balance within itself and with the universe. The medicine of ancient and medieval Western civilization is usually treated merely as the laughable ancestor of modern mechanical, biological, and chemical theories of medicine.[2] This book is therefore designed

humoral medicine:
Also known as humorism or humoralism, humoral medicine was the dominant medical theory in Europe and around the Mediterranean during classical antiquity and the Middle Ages. Humoral medicine is founded on the theory that the human body contains four vital liquids, or "humors": blood, phlegm, yellow bile, and black bile. These humors must be kept in balance to preserve good health. According to humoral theory, disease is caused by the excess or imbalance of certain humors. The creation of this theory is attributed to Hippocrates and it was elaborated in the following centuries by his many admirers, especially Galen.

---

1   For a concise introduction to all three medical systems, see William H. York, *Health and Wellness in Antiquity through the Middle Ages* (Greenwood, 2012). For more advanced studies on various humoral systems around the globe, see *The Body in Balance: Humoral Medicines in Practice*, edited by Peregrine Horden and Elisabeth Hsu (Berghahn, 2013), and *Knowledge and the Scholarly Medical Traditions*, edited by Don Bates (Cambridge UP, 1995). A valuable perspective on the essential differences between these traditions is given by Shigehisa Kuriyama, *The Expressiveness of the Body and the Divergence of Greek and Chinese Medicine* (Zone Books, 2002).

2   An important exception is the continued practice of Unani medicine of South Asia, which is based on the teachings of Ibn Sīnā (Avicenna), the most famous medieval Islamicate author on Hippocratic-Galenic medicine. See Documents 53 and 54, pp. 158–64.

to show both the significant continuities between premodern and modern medicine in Western culture and the contributions of multiple societies in Antiquity and the Middle Ages to the construction of this "Western medicine," including Ancient Egypt and Babylon, classical Greece and Rome, medieval Christian Europe and Byzantium, and the medieval **Islamicate** cultures of Spain, North Africa, and the Near East.

At the heart of humoral medicine is the theory that diseases are caused by an imbalance of four liquids, or humors, within the body: blood, phlegm, yellow or red bile, and black bile. The creation of this system is usually attributed to Hippocrates of Kos (ca. 460–370 BCE), but the identification of internal bodily fluids as the sources of disease was hardly original to the Greeks. Ancient Egyptians associated disease with corrupt or rotting substances within the body, called *wekhedu*, which had to be removed by purgation, especially through regular enemas. Likewise, Babylonian medicine emphasized the observation of bodily fluids to determine states of health or illness.

Egyptian or Babylonian medical theory, however, usually must be inferred, because the earliest medical writers did not describe their medical theories systematically and explicitly like the later Greeks. Hippocratic texts clearly express the idea that health is the state when the humors are in balance, or when an individual's dominant humor reigns peacefully over the others. Later Hippocratic physicians developed this theory further to argue that a person's dominant humor determined their "complexion" or "temperament," which refers to their entire physical and emotional disposition. This concept lies behind descriptions of people as sanguine (energetic and happy from blood, Latin *sanguis*), phlegmatic (relaxed and easy-going from phlegm, *phlegma*), choleric (ambitious or violent from red bile, *cholera*), or melancholic (introverted or sad from black bile, *melancholia*). This linguistic relic of premodern humoralism lasted even into the twentieth century, far longer than the actual medical system underlying it. Hippocrates' students and later admirers, especially Galen of Pergamon, promoted these aspects of Hippocratic medicine, so that "Hippocrates" eventually became synonymous with "humoralism."

Where modern medicine tends to describe our bodies like machines—a system of pumps and valves and pipes—premodern, humoral medicine is more organic, imagining the body as a container of constantly moving and interacting fluids. Hippocrates and his students developed this theory and, even though it faced competing medical systems in the ancient Mediterranean, it would come to prevail in medieval Jewish, Christian, and Islamic cultures. Hippocrates was as much a philosopher as a medical practitioner, and his approaches to understanding the causes of disease shaped Western medicine for the next 2,000 years. Nearly every primary

Islamicate: This word, coined by the historian of Islam Marshall Hodgson, is used throughout this collection to describe individuals and cultures which are not necessarily religiously Islamic, but are dominated culturally by Muslims. The term is useful because it includes not just Muslims, but any Christians, Jews, Zoroastrians, and Hindus who live under Islamic rule, and it includes languages other than Arabic which were used in those regions.

source in this volume is directly or indirectly shaped by the Hippocratic tradition of medicine.

This book is also designed to show the influence of religion on medicine (and the reverse) during Antiquity and the Middle Ages. Premodern Jews, Christians, and Muslims did not choose medicine *or* religion, as is sometimes popularly believed; rather, they were comfortable seeking both spiritual and natural cures for their ailments. Throughout this volume you will see evidence of healers invoking God or the gods to aid them in their diagnosis and treatment of diseases. While there was occasional tension between religion and natural medicine, usually they were mutually supportive and overlapping systems, so that by the end of the Middle Ages educated physicians could easily promote their faith and religious figures could teach and use the medicine of Hippocrates, Galen, and Avicenna.

HOW TO READ THIS COLLECTION

The documents in this volume reflect both the constancy of medical ideas in the premodern West and the diversity of local healing traditions underlying that constancy. They were written originally in ancient Egyptian, Babylonian, Greek, and Latin, as well as in Hebrew, Arabic, Judeo-Arabic (a term referring to several dialects and scripts used by Arabized Jews in the Middle Ages), medieval versions of Greek and Latin, and European vernaculars like Old English and Old French. All works are presented in modern English translations with occasional notes on the sense of words in the original languages. Some of these translations are recent, but others are one to two centuries old, and thus their language and tone (even in English) may seem difficult or bizarre to modern audiences. Students should remember that every generation of historians interprets and translates documents from the distant past in new ways, showing that history is an ongoing process of understanding rather than an unchanging set of facts.

The geographical and chronological scope of this work is designed to coincide with the first half of history survey sequences (Western Civilization or the West in the World) taught in many high schools and colleges. The documents are numbered from 1 to 91. A footnote to each source indicates the origin of the text and whether it is an existing translation or whether it is original to this volume. Every source is given a headnote explaining the author(s), date, and context of the work. Unfamiliar and interesting terms and ideas are explained with marginal annotations; these are indicated in **bold type**. The most common and important of these terms are also included in a Glossary at the end of the volume. Because there are hundreds of herbal ingredients mentioned in the ancient and medieval recipes below, most of them are not provided with annotations. The significance of the recipes is still clear without knowing the identity of every ingredient.

A note on transliteration of Arabic names: the Arabic letters *ayn* and *hamza* are both represented with a single straight quotation mark ['] for ease of reading. Long vowels are given macrons (e.g. ā) when that is the standard transliteration.

ABOUT THE COVER

The first document of this collection is found on the cover itself, a manuscript illumination from a late medieval medical manuscript of a work on anatomy falsely attributed to Galen. This dramatic figure is known to modern historians as a Wound Man, and is found frequently in European medical manuscripts and printed books from the later Middle Ages (fourteenth to sixteenth centuries). He belongs to a tradition of naked human figures that were labeled with medical information, including "bloodletting men" indicating the location of veins, pregnant women showing the development of the fetus, and "zodiac men" showing the influence of astrological signs on specific body parts (see Document 91, p. 262, for an example of a zodiac man). The Wound Man, although grievously injured by weapons, animal bites, and accidents, is still apparently alive. He stares out at us, using his naked body, labeled all around with Latin descriptions, to teach the art of medicine. Each wound is given a label on the outside and the locations of major organs are labeled on his inside. Physicians and surgeons used such an image not for treatment, but as a mnemonic device to remember the wide variety of injuries and wounds they might have to treat. He serves as a graphic reminder that, even though the collection below is composed mostly of extracts from books, the human body itself was the main text that a doctor should read.

CHRONOLOGY

Dates in this book are given with CE and BCE ("Common Era" and "Before the Common Era") which are the secular equivalent to the Christian dating system of AD and BC. When a date is given without CE or BCE, assume CE. The abbreviation "ca." means *circa*, Latin for "about." The following chronology includes many, but not all, of the major physicians, authors, and texts in this volume, along with a few key historical eras and events for context.

ca. 2650 BCE	Earliest named Egyptian physician
ca. 2400 BCE	Oldest Sumerian medical tablet
ca. 1820 BCE	Kahun Gynaecological Papyrus
ca. 1750 BCE	*Code of Hammurabi*
ca. 1550–ca. 1077 BCE	New Kingdom Egypt (time of most Egyptian medical papyri)
ca. 1200 BCE	Era of the Trojan War
ca. 750–650 BCE	Homeric poems written down
ca. 750–650 BCE	Hesiod
612 BCE	Library of Ashurbanipal destroyed
ca. 460–395 BCE	Thucydides
ca. 460–370 BCE	Hippocrates
430 BCE	Plague of Athens
428–348 BCE	Plato
ca. 400–300 BCE	Composition of most of the "Hippocratic Corpus"
384–322 BCE	Aristotle
371–287 BCE	Theophrastus
335–280 BCE	Herophilus
323 BCE	Death of Alexander the Great and start of "Hellenistic Era"

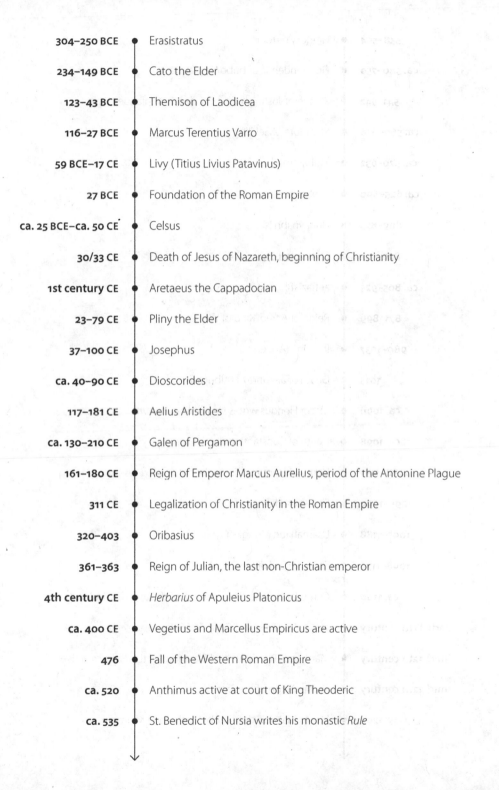

304–250 BCE	Erasistratus
234–149 BCE	Cato the Elder
123–43 BCE	Themison of Laodicea
116–27 BCE	Marcus Terentius Varro
59 BCE–17 CE	Livy (Titius Livius Patavinus)
27 BCE	Foundation of the Roman Empire
ca. 25 BCE–ca. 50 CE	Celsus
30/33 CE	Death of Jesus of Nazareth, beginning of Christianity
1st century CE	Aretaeus the Cappadocian
23–79 CE	Pliny the Elder
37–100 CE	Josephus
ca. 40–90 CE	Dioscorides
117–181 CE	Aelius Aristides
ca. 130–210 CE	Galen of Pergamon
161–180 CE	Reign of Emperor Marcus Aurelius, period of the Antonine Plague
311 CE	Legalization of Christianity in the Roman Empire
320–403	Oribasius
361–363	Reign of Julian, the last non-Christian emperor
4th century CE	*Herbarius* of Apuleius Platonicus
ca. 400 CE	Vegetius and Marcellus Empiricus are active
476	Fall of the Western Roman Empire
ca. 520	Anthimus active at court of King Theoderic
ca. 535	St. Benedict of Nursia writes his monastic *Rule*

538–594	Gregory of Tours
ca. 540–750	First Pandemic of bubonic plague
541–542	Plague of Justinian: First Pandemic of plague begins
ca. 560–636	St. Isidore of Seville
ca. 570–632	Muhammad
ca. 625–690	Paul of Aegina
809–873	Hunayn ibn Ishaq
820–912	Qustā ibn Lūqā
ca. 865–925	al-Rāzī (Rhazes)
871–899	Reign of Alfred, King of Wessex
980–1037	Ibn Sīnā (Avicenna)
1013	Death of al-Zahrawi (Albucasis)
ca. 1090	Macer Floridus writes *De viribus herbarum*
ca. 1098	Death of Constantine the African
ca. 1088–1157	Henry of Huntingdon, author of *Anglicanus Ortus*
1095–1099	First Crusade
1095–1188	Usamah ibn Munqidh
1098–1179	St. Hildegard of Bingen
ca. 1100	Compilation of *Articella* collection of Latin medical texts
early 12th century	Trota of Salerno and Copho of Salerno active
mid-12th century	Matthaeus Platearius and Platearius of the *Practica* active
mid-12th century	Composition of the *Trotula*
1135–1204	Moses Maimonides (Rabbi Moshe ben Maimon)

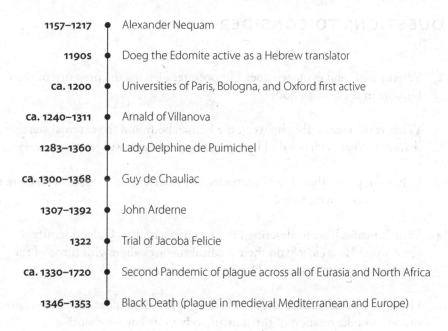

1157–1217	●	Alexander Nequam
1190s	●	Doeg the Edomite active as a Hebrew translator
ca. 1200	●	Universities of Paris, Bologna, and Oxford first active
ca. 1240–1311	●	Arnald of Villanova
1283–1360	●	Lady Delphine de Puimichel
ca. 1300–1368	●	Guy de Chauliac
1307–1392	●	John Arderne
1322	●	Trial of Jacoba Felicie
ca. 1330–1720	●	Second Pandemic of plague across all of Eurasia and North Africa
1346–1353	●	Black Death (plague in medieval Mediterranean and Europe)

QUESTIONS TO CONSIDER

1. What proofs and evidence does Hippocrates give for the presence of the four humors in the human body?

2. What is the relationship between the human body and the external weather and seasons? What evidence do Hippocrates and other classical authors provide?

3. What symptoms does Hippocrates look at to diagnose diseases? What are the causes of those symptoms?

4. Which medical "sects" described in Document 19 does Galen identify most with? How closely do their medical theories align with those of the Hippocratic Corpus seen in Documents 7 and 10–13?

5. How did epidemics and plagues challenge prevailing ideas about the causes of disease and the relation of the human body to its environment?

6. Study the selections from Dioscorides' *De materia medica* in Document 23. What aspects of the plant or its healing abilities does he focus on in each entry? How does this compare with medieval descriptions of medicinal plants in Documents 37–40 and 73–75?

7. What were the abilities and expectations of the gods in relation to healing? Compare Asclepius with the one God of the Jews, Christian, and Muslims.

8. How could the idea of "complexion" be applied to both people and plants or food? What does this say about medieval physicians' understanding of nature?

9. What aspects of Hippocratic-Galenic medicine did medieval Islamicate and European physicians find most appealing?

10. Were medieval physicians able to fit their explanations of specific diseases or conditions (Documents 58–59 and 66–68) into the dominant medical theory, or did they start changing their theory to match the diseases?

11. How were women seen as inherently different from men in medieval medicine? How did this affect diagnosis and treatment?

12. How can a modern historian identify "magical" elements in medieval medical practice? Why was astrology not considered magic at that time?

PART 1

The Earliest Medical Writings of the Near East and Mediterranean (ca. 2000–700 BCE)

Western medicine before Hippocrates in the fifth century BCE is often called "pre-rational" or "irrational," to highlight the differences between the frequently supernatural remedies typically found in ancient Egyptian and Mesopotamian medical writings, and the naturalism and apparent rationality of the Hippocratic medical writings.[1] "Irrational" means that the earliest medical authors often attribute the causes of disease to gods, spirits, demons, or ancestors, and seek cures through religious or magical rituals. These are explanations and activities that are explicitly rejected in Hippocratic writings. A favorite example used by historians to highlight this difference is the case of epilepsy. The Mesopotamian medical text known as the *Sakikku* (Akkadian language, 1067–1046 BCE) states that epileptic fits are caused by possession by a demon or departed spirit. By comparison, the Hippocratic work *On the Sacred Disease* (ca. 400 BCE) emphasizes the natural origin of epileptic fits through an excess of phlegm in the brain and explicitly rejects divine or supernatural causes.

There is no doubting the important differences between the earliest healing systems of Western civilization and those of the classical Greeks and Romans. However, we must be careful not to overemphasize the differences, for Egyptian and Mesopotamian physicians were practicing for 2,000 and more years before Hippocrates, and recording significant medical observations alongside their supernatural remedies. Physicians and healers are described in some of the world's earliest documents in Egypt and Mesopotamia. Hesy-Ra is the first named physician (*swnw* in Egyptian), dating from the 3rd Dynasty of the Old Kingdom, around 2650 BCE. For the next millennium, numerous other physicians appear in the written record and tombs, but we know little of their medical practice. We have to

---

1 For example, see James Longrigg, *Greek Medicine from the Heroic to the Hellenistic Age: A Source Book* (Routledge, 1998), 5.

wait until the second millennium BCE for the survival of clearly medical documents, all of which are written on papyrus, and so are usually known as the "medical papyri."

The oldest Egyptian medical text, and possibly the oldest medical document in the world, is the "Kahun Gynaecological Papyrus" of ca. 1820 BCE (Document 1). Historians consider it properly "medical" because it provides descriptions of human ailments and instructions for their treatment and cure, in this case, mostly conditions related to pregnancy and childbirth. The longest of the ancient Egyptian medical papyri is the "Ebers Papyrus" from 1534 BCE (Document 2), which includes over 700 formulas, spells, and recipes. Both the Kahun and Ebers papyri are written in the form of instructions to doctors, indicating how they should address the patient, identify the disease or injury, and prescribe a medicine or treatment. Such medical papyri may have been intended for the education of new doctors, who needed practice in developing an authoritative and comforting bedside manner.

Ancient Mesopotamians, like the Egyptians, made little or no distinction between magic, religion, and medicine when it came to treatment. All means were available for healing a patient, including incantations, prayer, pharmacological substances, dietary changes, massage, and fumigations. The roles of physician and priest frequently overlapped for both the diagnosis and cure of diseases. Most Mesopotamian medical literature survives in the form of clay tablets written in cuneiform script, but in different languages like Sumerian, Akkadian, or Babylonian. Some 660 of the approximately 1,000 surviving Mesopotamian medical tablets come from the library of Ashurbanipal, king of Nineveh (r. 668–627 BCE). Ashurbanipal was a great collector of all forms of earlier Mesopotamian literature, from mathematics and medicine to the *Epic of Gilgamesh*. Some of the tablets of Ashurbanipal are considered faithful copies of much older documents. Invaders destroyed the library in 612 BCE, but most of the clay tablets survived and were discovered by archeologists in 1853. One of those tablets includes a series of Babylonian spells against fever, found below in Document 3.

Roughly contemporary with the Babylonian medical spell are some of the earliest Greek writings which mention disease, injury, and healing (Documents 4–6). These Greek sources are not strictly medical, like the previously discussed Egyptian and Babylonian sources, but come rather from the epic poems of Homer and Hesiod. The Homeric *Iliad* and *Odyssey* were written down in the eighth and seventh centuries BCE but draw on Mycenaean oral traditions of several centuries earlier around the time of the semi-legendary Trojan War in the thirteenth century BCE. The poems are typically attributed to the same person, "Homer," but were probably the product of at least two different poets who synthesized generations of oral poetry. The Homeric poems feature many instances of wounding and sickness, which are treated variously by soldiers, priests, or doctors (Document 6). In fact, the *Iliad* begins with a plague sent by the god Apollo, which devastates the Greek troops as they besiege the city of Troy (Document 4). Both the disease and the cure are given religious explanations, a theme which will reoccur in times of plague throughout Antiquity and the Middle Ages (see Documents 26, p. 86, and 46–48, pp. 134–40) alongside natural explanations. Hesiod (ca. 750–650 BCE) was a contemporary of Homer who wrote several didactic poems intended for teaching his fellow Greeks about the gods, agriculture, morals, and good economics. His most important works are the *Theogony* and *Works and Days*, the latter of which explains in religious terms why people get sick and particularly why entire communities fall ill from epidemic disease (Document 5).

DOCUMENT 1:

The Kahun Gynaecological Papyrus[2]

The Kahun Papyrus, written about 1820 BCE, contains fragments of 34
separate recipes, all intended for women, and especially for treating conditions
of the uterus and vulva and for determining or preventing conception. It
is indicative of the importance of women having healthy pregnancies and
childbirth for any society that the world's earliest surviving medical document
is dedicated to this subject. This document is directed to the physician and
provides a script for questioning the patient and explaining the disease and
treatment.

ৎ৶

1. Treatment for a woman whose eyes ache who sees not; and has pain in
the neck. *Thou shalt say as to it:* "It is excretions from the womb, in her eyes."
Thou shalt do for it thus: **fumigate** her on incense and fresh fat; fumigate her
vagina with this; fumigate her eyes with the shanks of the legs of **bee-eaters**;
thou shalt make her eat the liver of an ass, raw.

2. Treatment for a woman suffering in her womb from walking. *Thou shalt
say as to it:* "What is the smell thou emittest?" If she says to thee, "I am
emitting the smell of roast meat," *thou shalt say as to it,* it is a disorder of the
womb. *Thou shalt do for it thus:* fumigate her with every sort of roast meat,
the smell of which she emits.

3. Treatment for a woman pained in her buttocks, her abdomen, and the
backs of her thighs. *Thou shalt say as to it:* "It is excretions of the womb." *Thou
shalt do for it thus:* carob beans 1/64 *hekt*; *shasha* fruit 1/64 *hekt*; cow's milk 1
henu; cook, cool, make into one mass, drink four mornings.

4. Treatment for a woman on her belly, her vagina, the parts which surround
her vagina, and within her kidneys. *Thou shalt say as to it:* "It is the being
made very big of the fetus." *Thou shalt do for it thus:* fresh fat 1 *henu:* spread
in her vagina in....

fumigate: The burning of
a substance for medical
purposes, to be inhaled or
brought up into the uterus.

bee-eaters: A genus of
insectivorous birds in Africa
and the Near East. They
were the subject of folklore
and medicine in several
ancient cultures.

---

2   *The Petrie Papyri. Hieratic Papyri from Kahun and Gurob (Principally of the Middle Kingdom),* edited
by F.L. Griffith (London, 1898), 6–7. Modified.

DOCUMENT 2:

Diagnosis in Ancient Egypt: The Ebers Papyrus[3]

> The Ebers Papyrus, dated to 1534 BCE, contains the most extensive record of ancient Egyptian medicine, containing equal doses of pathology (disease identification) and therapeutics, both magical and rational in character. The passage below takes the form of instructions to the doctor for identifying internal abdominal medical conditions. Each item includes a description of an ailment, an authoritative statement for the doctor to make to the patient or others in attendance, and instructions for preparing and administering the herbal remedies. The diseases are not given specific names but are described as sets of symptoms. No causes, natural or otherwise, are given for these medical conditions.

ε

1. When thou examinest a person who suffers from an obstruction in his abdomen and thou findest that it goes-and-comes under the fingers like oil-in-a-tube, then say thou: "It all comes from his mouth like slime!"

Prepare for him: Fruit-of-the-Dompalm, Dissolve in Man's Semen, Crush, cook in Oil and Honey.

To be eaten by the Patient for four mornings. Afterwards let him be smeared with dried, crushed, and pressed maqut grain.

2. When thou examinest the obstruction in his abdomen and thou findest that he is not in a condition to leap the Nile, his stomach is swollen and his chest asthmatic, then say thou to him "It is the Blood that has got itself fixed and does not circulate." Do thou cause an emptying by means of a medicinal remedy.

Make him therefore: Wormwood 1/8, Elderberries 1/16, sebesten 1/8, sasa-chips 1/8.

Cook in Beer-that-has-been-brewed-from-many-ingredients, strain into one, thoroughly, and let the Patient drink.

3. This remedy drives out blood through his mouth or rectum which resembles Hog's Blood when-it-is-cooked. Either make him a poultice to cool

---

3   Cyril P. Brian, *The Papyrus Ebers, Translated from the German Version* (D. Appleton & Co., 1931).

him in front, or thou dost not prepare him this remedy, but makest for him the following really excellent Ointment composed of: Ox fat, Saffron seeds, Coriander, Myrrh, aager-tree.

Crush and apply as a poultice.

4. When thou examinest a person who has a hardening, his stomach hurts him, his face is pale, his heart thumps; when thou examinest him and findest his heart and stomach burning and his body swollen, then it is the *sexen*-illness in the Depths and the fire is consuming him. Make him a remedy that quenches the fire and empties his bowels by drinking Sweet-Beer-that-has-stood-in-dry-Dough. This is to be eaten and drunk for four days. Look every morning for six days following at what falls from his rectum. If excrement falls out of him like little black lumps, then say to him: "The body-fire has fallen from the stomach. The asi-disease in the body has diminished." If thou examinest him after this has come to pass and something steps forth from his rectum like the white of beans and drops shoot forth out of him like nesu-of-tepaut, then thou sayest: "What was in his abdomen has fallen down." MAKE FOR HIM THIS REMEDY SO THAT HIS FACE MAY COOL. Stand the cauldron over the fire, make a mixture in it and cook it in the usual way.

TO DRIVE AWAY THE HARDENING IN THE ABDOMEN: Bread-of-the-Zizyphus-Lotus, 1; Watermelon, 1; Cat's dung, 1; Sweet Beer, 1; Wine, 1.

Make into one and apply as a poultice.

DOCUMENT 3:

A Babylonian Spell against Fever[4]

This healing spell was recorded on a clay tablet in the library of Ashurbanipal of Nineveh. It was inscribed during the seventh century BCE but probably reflects medical traditions going back to the Sumerians in the third millennium BCE. The spell comes from an important series of tablets that are both medical and religious in nature, as they include ritual treatments for *Asakku*, a term which includes both fevers and divine curses. Whereas many treatments for *Asakku* are spells against demons, those found on the "Fever Sickness" tablets (*Asakki Marsuti*) seem to describe a more obvious physical condition like a fever.

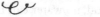

Incantation:

Fever unto the man, against his head, hath drawn nigh,
Disease unto the man, against his life, hath drawn nigh,
An evil Spirit against his neck hath drawn nigh,
An evil Demon against his breast hath drawn nigh,
An evil ghost against his belly hath drawn nigh,
An evil Devil against his hand hath drawn nigh,
An evil God against his foot hath drawn nigh,
These seven together have seized upon him,
His body like a consuming fire they devour,
As one that worketh evil they have ... him,
As with a garment they envelop him....

Marduk hath seen him: (etc.),
"What I": (etc.),
"Go, my son, take a dark-coloured kid whose stomach hath been taken away. A fat lamb whose leg hath been taken away. Thou shalt flay off the skin, thou shalt tear away the ...
Hand and foot an image ... thou shalt set the sick man ... thou shalt place....

"That the great gods may remove the evil,
That the evil Spirit may stand aside,
May the evil Spirit, the evil Demon stand aside,

---

4   R. Campbell Thompson, *The Devils and Evil Spirits of Babylonia*, 2 vols. (London, 1903–04), Vol. 2, 29–37. Modified.

May a kindly Spirit, a kindly Genius be present."

Incantation:

Fever hath blown upon the man as the windblast,
It hath smitten this man, and humbled his pride,
It hath smitten his ... and hath brought him low,
It hath rotted his thews like a girdle,
His mouth it hath turned to gall
So that the moisture therein hath no sweetness,
... so that he cannot move his limbs,
[five or more lines are destroyed here]

The man can eat no food, no water can he drink,
He cannot sleep, he hath no rest,
His god hath let him be brought low.

Marduk hath seen him: (etc.),
"What I": (etc.),
"Go, my son, take a white kid of Tammuz, lay it down facing the sick man and take out its heart and place it in the hand of that man. Perform the Incantation of Eridu, the kid whose heart thou hast taken out is **li'i-food** with which thou shalt make an atonement for the man. Bring forth a censer and a torch, scatter it in the street, bind a bandage on that man, perform the Incantation of Eridu, invoke the great gods that the evil Spirit, the evil Demon, evil Ghost, Hag-demon, Ghoul, Fever, or heavy Sickness which is in the body of the man, may be removed and go forth from the house! May a kindly Spirit, a kindly Genius be present!"

O evil Spirit! O evil Demon! O evil Ghost! O Hag-demon! O Ghoul! O Sickness of the heart! O Heartache! O Headache! O Toothache! O Pestilence! O grievous Fever! By Heaven and Earth may ye be exorcised!

li'i-food: It is unclear what *li'i* are exactly, but given the context they are surely some kind of evil spirits that must be appeased with the sacrificed goat kid.

DOCUMENT 4:

Plague as Divine Punishment in Homer's *Iliad* I: 1–119[5]

> Homer's *Iliad*, written down in the eighth or seventh century BCE, opens
> with a scene of disease and healing, during the tenth year of the war between
> the Greeks and the Trojans. The god Apollo punishes the invading Achaeans
> (Greeks) with a plague for dishonoring his priest (not the bubonic plague,
> which was caused by *Yersinia pestis*). This plague, inflicted by a god for
> religious reasons, could thus only be averted and cured by religious means.

e

Sing, O goddess, the anger of Achilles son of Peleus, that brought countless
ills upon the Achaeans. Many a brave soul did it send hurrying down to
Hades, and many a hero did it yield a prey to dogs and vultures, for so were
the counsels of Jove fulfilled from the day on which the son of Atreus, king
of men, and great Achilles, first fell out with one another.

And which of the gods was it that set them on to quarrel? It was the son
of Jove and Leto; for he was angry with the king and sent a pestilence upon
the host to plague the people, because the son of Atreus had dishonoured
Chryses his priest. Now Chryses had come to the ships of the Achaeans to
free his daughter, and had brought with him a great ransom: moreover he
bore in his hand the sceptre of Apollo wreathed with a suppliant's wreath
and he besought the Achaeans, but most of all the two sons of Atreus, who
were their chiefs.

"Sons of Atreus," he cried, "and all other Achaeans, may the gods who
dwell in Olympus grant you to sack the city of Priam, and to reach your
homes in safety; but free my daughter, and accept a ransom for her, in
reverence to Apollo, son of Jove."

On this the rest of the Achaeans with one voice were for respecting the
priest and taking the ransom that he offered; but not so Agamemnon, who
spoke fiercely to him and sent him roughly away. "Old man," said he, "let
me not find you tarrying about our ships, nor yet coming hereafter. Your
sceptre of the god and your wreath shall profit you nothing. I will not free
her. She shall grow old in my house at Argos far from her own home, busying
herself with her loom and visiting my couch; so go, and do not provoke me
or it shall be the worse for you."

The old man feared him and obeyed. Not a word he spoke, but went
by the shore of the sounding sea and prayed apart to King Apollo whom

---

5   *The Iliad of Homer, Rendered into English Prose*, translated by Samuel Butler (Longman, Green, and
     Co., 1898).

lovely Leto had borne. "Hear me," he cried, "O god of the silver bow, that protectest Chryse and holy Cilla and rulest Tenedos with thy might, hear me oh thou of Sminthe. If I have ever decked your temple with garlands, or burned your thigh-bones in fat of bulls or goats, grant my prayer, and let your arrows avenge these my tears upon the Danaans."

Thus did he pray, and Apollo heard his prayer. He came down furious from the summits of Olympus, with his bow and his quiver upon his shoulder, and the arrows rattled on his back with the rage that trembled within him. He sat himself down away from the ships with a face as dark as night, and his silver bow rang death as he shot his arrow in the midst of them. First he smote their mules and their hounds, but presently he aimed his shafts at the people themselves, and all day long the pyres of the dead were burning.

For nine whole days he shot his arrows among the people, but upon the tenth day Achilles called them in assembly—moved thereto by Juno, who saw the Achaeans in their death-throes and had compassion upon them. Then, when they were got together, he rose and spoke among them.

"Son of Atreus," said he, "I deem that we should now turn roving home if we would escape destruction, for we are being cut down by war and pestilence at once. Let us ask some priest or prophet, or some reader of dreams (for dreams, too, are of Jove) who can tell us why Phoebus Apollo is so angry, and say whether it is for some vow that we have broken, or hecatomb that we have not offered, and whether he will accept the savour of lambs and goats without blemish, so as to take away the plague from us."

DOCUMENT 5:

Gods as the Source of Disease: Hesiod, *Works and Days*[6]

Homer's contemporary Hesiod (ca. 750–650 BCE) also understood diseases as willed by the gods. In his didactic poem *Works and Days*, he paints a dreary picture of humanity, constantly beset by diseases, some of which are specifically sent by Zeus ("son of Cronos") to punish whole cities for the sins of even one bad man. Unlike Homer, Hesiod does not describe any cure (natural or religious) for these diseases—they are simply the fate of all people.

❧

For ere this the tribes of men lived on earth remote and free from ills and hard toil and heavy sicknesses which bring the Fates upon men; for in misery men grow old quickly. But the woman took off the great lid of the jar with her hands and scattered, all these and her thought caused sorrow and mischief to men. Only Hope remained there in an unbreakable home within under the rim of the great jar, and did not fly out at the door; for ere that, the lid of the jar stopped her, by the will of Aegis-holding Zeus who gathers the clouds. But the rest, countless plagues, wander amongst men; for earth is full of evils, and the sea is full. Of themselves diseases come upon men continually by day and by night, bringing mischief to mortals silently; for wise Zeus took away speech from them. So is there no way to escape the will of Zeus. Or if you will, I will sum you up another tale well and skilfully—and do you lay it up in your heart,—how the gods and mortal men sprang from one source.

... But for those who practice violence and cruel deeds far-seeing Zeus, the son of Cronos, ordains a punishment. Often even a whole city suffers for a bad man who sins and devises presumptuous deeds, and the son of Cronos lays great trouble upon the people, famine and plague together, so that the men perish away, and their women do not bear children, and their houses become few, through the contriving of Olympian Zeus. And again, at another time, the son of Cronos either destroys their wide army, or their walls, or else makes an end of their ships on the sea. You princes, mark well this punishment, you also, for the deathless gods are near among men; and mark all those who oppress their fellows with crooked judgements; and heed not the anger of the gods. For upon the bounteous earth Zeus has thrice ten thousand spirits, watchers of mortal men, and these keep watch on judgements and deeds of wrong as they roam, clothed in mist, all over the earth.

---

6   Hesiod, *Works and Days*, in *The Homeric Hymns and Homerica*, translated by Hugh G. Evelyn-White (Macmillan, 1914), lines 90–108, 238–56.

DOCUMENT 6:

Violence and Healing in Homeric Greece[7]

Homer's *Iliad* and *Odyssey* include so many details of anatomy, the effects of violent wounds, and their treatments that some modern scholars have proposed that Homer himself was a physician. There is no way of knowing that for sure, but these passages from his *Iliad* show graphically how ancient Greeks could gauge the depth and severity of a wound received in battle. Unlike the religious cures for the divinely sent plague in Document 4, pp. 19–20, these wounds are treated by surgery and painkilling herbs.

ლ

Menelaos Is Struck by an Arrow and Treated by the Healer Machaon (Homer, *Iliad* IV: 127–219)

But the blessed gods did not forget you, O Menelaos, and Zeus' daughter, driver of the spoil, was the first to stand before you and ward off the piercing arrow. She turned it from his skin as a mother whisks a fly from off her child when it is sleeping sweetly; she guided it to the part where the golden buckles of the belt that passed over his double **cuirass** were fastened, so the arrow struck the belt that went tightly round him. It went right through this and through the cuirass of cunning workmanship; it also pierced the belt beneath it, which he wore next his skin to keep out darts or arrows; it was this that served him in the best stead, nevertheless the arrow went through it and grazed the top of the skin, so that blood began flowing from the wound....

When King Agamemnon saw the blood flowing from the wound he was afraid, and so was brave Menelaos himself till he saw that the barbs of the arrow and the thread that bound the arrow-head to the shaft were still outside the wound. Then he took heart, but Agamemnon heaved a deep sigh as he held Menelaos' hand in his own, and his comrades made moan in concert....

But Menelaos reassured him and said, "Take heart, and do not alarm the people; the arrow has not struck me in a mortal part, for my outer belt of burnished metal first stayed it, and under this my cuirass and the belt of mail which the bronze-smiths made me." And Agamemnon answered, "I trust, dear Menelaos, that it may be even so, but the surgeon shall examine your wound and lay herbs upon it to relieve your pain."

- **cuirass:** A piece of armor, usually formed of a breastplate and backplate together.

---

7 *The Iliad of Homer, Rendered into English Prose*, translated by Samuel Butler (London, 1898).

He then said to Talthybios, "Talthybios, tell Machaon, son to the great physician, Asklepios,[8] to come and see Menelaos immediately. Some Trojan or Lycian archer has wounded him with an arrow to our dismay, and to his own great glory."

Talthybios did as he was told, and went about the host trying to find Machaon. Presently he found him standing amid the brave warriors who had followed him from Tricca; thereon he went up to him and said, "Son of Asklepios, King Agamemnon says you are to come and see Menelaos immediately. Some Trojan or Lycian archer has wounded him with an arrow to our dismay and to his own great glory."

Thus did he speak, and Machaon was moved to go. They passed through the spreading host of the Achaeans and went on till they came to the place where Menelaos had been wounded and was lying with the chieftains gathered in a circle round him. Machaon passed into the middle of the ring and at once drew the arrow from the belt, bending its barbs back through the force with which he pulled it out. He undid the burnished belt, and beneath this the cuirass and the belt of mail which the bronze-smiths had made; then, when he had seen the wound, he wiped away the blood and applied some soothing drugs which Chiron had given to Asklepios out of the good will he bore him.

Anatomical Observation of a Deadly Injury (Homer, *Iliad* XIII: 640–59)

So saying Menelaos stripped the blood-stained armour from the body of Pisander, and handed it over to his men; then he again ranged himself among those who were in the front of the fight. Harpalion son of King Pylaemenes then sprang upon him; he had come to fight at Troy along with his father, but he did not go home again. He struck the middle of Menelaos's shield with his spear but could not pierce it, and to save his life drew back under cover of his men, looking round him on every side lest he should be wounded. But Meriones aimed a bronze-tipped arrow at him as he was leaving the field, and hit him on the right buttock; the arrow pierced the bone through and through, and penetrated the bladder, so he sat down where he was and breathed his last in the arms of his comrades, stretched like a worm upon the ground and watering the earth with the blood that flowed from his wound. The brave Paphlagonians tended him with all due care; they raised him into his chariot, and bore him sadly off to the city of Troy; his father went also with him weeping bitterly, but there was no ransom that could bring his dead son to life again.

---

8   See Documents 13–18, pp. 52–61, about the centaur Chiron and healing god Asklepios (Asclepius).

Medicine and Healing among the Ancient Greeks (ca. 500 BCE–200 CE)

RATIONAL MEDICINE IN THE AGE OF HIPPOCRATES (DOCUMENTS 7–12)

Histories of medicine frequently begin with Hippocrates of Kos (ca. 460–370 BCE), and with good reason. The so-called father of Western medicine is celebrated for bringing systematic reasoning to the practice of medicine, arguing that diseases have natural and rational—as opposed to supernatural and arbitrary—causes, which can be determined by studying the patient's symptoms, environment, diet, and lifestyle. This approach to healing underlies many of the documents in this collection. The documents in the first half of Part 2 thus focus on classical Greek medical theory, the ideas developed to explain or support medical practice. These include several works by Hippocrates or by his students and followers, by the philosopher Plato, and by their contemporary, the historian Thucydides.

Documents 1 to 6 above demonstrate that ancient doctors did practice detailed observation of symptoms and the diagnosis of disease many centuries before Hippocrates, even if they did not clearly separate supernatural and natural causes. What, then, was different about the classical Greeks in general, and Hippocrates in particular? For one thing, Greeks during the sixth and fifth centuries BCE, the beginning of the Classical Era, wrote and disputed extensively about the natural (rather than divine or supernatural) causes of phenomena in the world around them. These phenomena included pain, disease, and bodily functions, which philosophers and physicians discussed using sophisticated reasoning, exploratory arguments, and specific criticisms of other authors or teachers.

Even before Hippocrates, medical texts were widespread in Greek and Ionian cities and they reflect different schools of thought about nature and the human body. The earliest of the Hippocratic texts, some perhaps by Hippocrates himself, throw us into an already active public debate about how medicine should be practiced. For example, the Hippocratic work called *The Art of Medicine* defends medicine against its detractors, while another called *Ancient Medicine* criticizes those who overly philosophize medicine. Despite this criticism, many classical Greek philosophers had something to say about medicine, disease, or human physiology. Pythagoras and his followers, for example, refused to eat meat, fish, or beans (although probably for religious rather than medical reasons) and the Pythagorean focus on numbers as the foundation of the cosmos may have lent support to the later classical and medieval doctrine of "critical days" during an illness.[1]

Many physicians practiced and some wrote about medicine in classical Greece, but most of their ideas have been lost, in part because Hippocrates came to be almost the sole name in the investigation of disease and the practice of rational medicine during the Hellenistic period (ca. 300–31 BCE). This is why the name of Hippocrates now graces some 60 different Greek medical treatises written between the fifth and first centuries BCE by Hippocrates himself, his students, and later imitators and admirers; these works are known collectively as the "Hippocratic Corpus." Historians of ancient medicine still debate vigorously which works are genuinely by Hippocrates, but for our purposes it is important to understand that later Roman and medieval scholars considered nearly every work attributed to "Hippocrates" to be genuine.

The Hippocratics wrote about many medical topics, but are best known for analyzing the nature and causes of disease. This is evident in the treatise *Nature of Man* (Document 7), which includes one of the earliest systematic descriptions of the four humors as part of human physiology, health, and disease. A less systematic work, but one which might more accurately reflect the real Hippocrates' teaching, is the *Aphorisms*, a collection of brief and enigmatic statements about medical learning and practice (Document 10). The first aphorism is one of the most famous statements in Hippocratic medicine, laying out succinctly how difficult it is both to learn the entire art of medicine and to make correct judgments in diagnosis and treatment: "Life is short, and Art long; the crisis fleeting; experience perilous, and decision difficult." Physicians today are still confronted with these same problems: How can we balance the apparently endless amount of medical learning with the immediate desire to heal? How do we negotiate between a universalizing science of medicine and the personal needs of an individual patient?

Another classical Greek who rationally investigated the causes of disease was Plato (ca. 428–348 BCE). Plato is today better known for his political and moral philosophy, but he also observed and wrote about contemporary Greek medicine in his dialogue *Timaeus* (Document 8). Our best contemporary

---

1   Vivian Nutton, *Ancient Medicine*, 2nd ed. (Routledge, 2013), 43–46.

evidence for Hippocrates himself comes from Plato, who mentions him in his dialogues *Phaedrus* and *Protagoras*. Plato assumed that Hippocrates is well known to his audience and calls him an "Asclepiad," a follower of, or someone who claimed to be a descendant of, the demi-god Asclepius himself (see Documents 13–18, pp. 52–61). In classical Greece, it was not just physicians like Hippocrates or philosophers like Plato who explored rational and natural causes of human phenomena, but also historians like Thucydides (460–395 BCE). Thucydides was a soldier and general for the *polis* (city-state) of Athens. He survived both the war and the plague which struck Athens in 430 BCE (not bubonic plague, but possibly typhus or typhoid fever). In his *History of the Peloponnesian War* (Document 9), Thucydides describes the plague's progress, symptoms, and effects, but does not explore its cause. His wholly natural and human description of the disease influenced Western descriptions of other plagues for the next two millennia. When Byzantine Greek authors tried to describe the devastation of the First Pandemic of bubonic plague in the sixth and seventh centuries CE (see Document 46, pp. 135–36), they turned immediately to Thucydides as a rhetorical model.

Most Hippocratic medicine was non-invasive: treatments were based primarily on increasing or restricting the diet (*diaita*).[2] This "diet" was not just food and drink, but also included exercise, bathing, and sexual activity, as can be seen in the Hippocratic treatises *Regimen* and *Airs, Waters, Places*, the latter of which is excerpted in Document 11. These works teach that a patient is a product of his or her environment and that the best physician must understand that environment to properly treat the individual, ideas which have only come back into modern Western medicine in the last few decades. This "holistic" approach to healing informed much of Greco-Roman and medieval medicine, as can be seen in later examples of medical regimens in Documents 22 and 63 (pp. 76–77 and 191–94).

Ancient Greece had a similar diversity of healers to ancient Egypt or Babylon, but it was Greek culture in particular that set up on a pedestal the learned physician (Greek *iatros*, from which we get "psychiatry," "pediatrician," "geriatric"). The physician was distinguished from the barber (who also pulled teeth) or surgeon by his focus on diagnosis (identifying the nature of a disease) and prognosis (determining a disease's outcome). Without any of the tools of a modern laboratory, the most an ancient physician usually could do was to watch the patient and ask them pointed questions. We see this behavior modeled in the Hippocratic *Epidemics* (Document 12). The author provides detailed descriptions of the symptoms and outcome (usually death)

---

2   Jacques Jouanna, "Dietetics in Hippocratic medicine: Definition, main problems, discussion," in *Greek Medicine from Hippocrates to Galen: Selected Papers*, edited by Philip van der Eijk and translated by Neil Allies (Brill, 2012), 137–53.

of a variety of Greek patients suffering from some sort of feverish epidemic disease. He does this to provide particular cases by which the learned physician can develop a judgment of the universal nature of certain diseases. This movement from the particular to the universal is central to the development of ancient philosophy, especially that associated with Aristotle. The narrator makes no attempt to cure or intervene, but only observes: this is a teaching document. Likewise, the Hippocratic author is not concerned with naming a specific disease, but rather with detailing the progress of symptoms so that students can learn to make accurate prognoses themselves.

DOCUMENT 7:

Hippocratic Corpus, *Nature of Man*[3]

> The Hippocratic treatise *Nature of Man* includes one of the earliest systematic descriptions of the humors as part of human physiology, health, and disease. It might have been written by Hippocrates' student and son-in-law, Polybius, during the fourth century BCE but it probably reflects original Hippocratic teachings of the fifth century. One of the reasons given by historians for this early date is that the author does not clearly state that there are four distinct humors and, at times, he treats yellow bile and black bile simply as two versions of the single humor "bile." This lack of clarity on black bile will return in Galen's work on the subject below in Document 25, pp. 83–85.

॒

IV. The body of man has in itself **blood**, **phlegm**, yellow bile and black bile; these make up the nature of his body, and through these he feels pain or enjoys health. Now he enjoys the most perfect health when these **elements** are duly proportioned to one another in respect of compounding, power and bulk, and when they are perfectly mingled. Pain is felt when one of these elements is in defect or excess, or is isolated in the body without being compounded with all the others. For when an element is isolated and stands by itself, not only must the place which it left become diseased, but the place where it stands in a **flood** must, because of the excess, cause pain and distress. In fact when more of an element flows out of the body than is necessary to get rid of superfluity, the emptying causes pain. If, on the other hand, it be to an inward part that there takes place the emptying, the shifting and the separation from other elements, the man certainly must, according to what has been said, suffer from a double pain, one in the place left, and another in the place flooded.

V. Now I promised to show that what are according to me the constituents of man remain always the same, according to both convention and nature. These constituents are, I hold, blood, phlegm, yellow bile and black bile. First I assert that the names of these according to convention are separated, and that none of them has the same name as the others; furthermore, that according to nature their essential forms are separated, phlegm being quite unlike blood, blood being quite unlike bile, bile being quite unlike phlegm. How could they be like one another, when their colors appear not alike

blood: In premodern Western medicine blood (Latin *sanguis* and Greek *haema*) could refer both to the pure humor of blood, representing the hot and moist qualities of the body, or the blood that flows through the veins, which is a composite of all four humors. Context is necessary to determine which *sanguis* the author intended.

phlegm: One of the four primary humors of humoral medicine, representing the cold and moist qualities of the body. The mucus we now call phlegm is only one manifestation of this essential humor.

elements: "Element" here should be understood as one of the four bodily humors and not as one of the four classical elements of earth, air, fire, and water.

flood: When the element is in dangerous excess.

---

3 *Hippocrates*, Vol. IV, edited and translated by W.H.S. Jones (William Heinemann, 1931), 11–15, 19–29.

to the sight nor does their touch seem alike to the hand? For they are not equally warm, nor cold, nor dry, nor moist. Since then they are so different from one another in essential form and in power, they cannot be one, if fire and water are not one. From the following evidence you may know that these elements are not all one, but that each of them has its own power and its own nature. If you were to give a man a medicine which withdraws phlegm, he will vomit you phlegm; if you give him one which withdraws bile, he will vomit you bile. Similarly too black bile is purged away if you give a medicine which withdraws black bile. And if you wound a man's body so as to cause a wound, blood will flow from him. And you will find all these things happen on any day and on any night, both in winter and in summer, so long as the man can draw breath in and then breathe it out again, or until he is deprived of one of the elements congenital with him....

VII. Phlegm increases in a man in winter; for phlegm, being the coldest constituent of the body, is closest akin to winter. A proof that phlegm is very cold is that if you touch phlegm, bile and blood, you will find phlegm the coldest. And yet it is the most viscid, and after black bile requires most force for its evacuation. But things that are moved by force become hotter under the stress of the force. Yet in spite of all this, phlegm shows itself the coldest element by reason of its own nature. That winter fills the body with phlegm you can learn from the following evidence. It is in winter that the **sputum** and nasal discharge of men is fullest of phlegm; at this season mostly swellings become white, and diseases generally phlegmatic. And in spring too phlegm still remains strong in the body, while the blood increases. For the cold relaxes, and the rains come on, while the blood accordingly increases through the showers and the hot days. For these conditions of the year are most akin to the nature of blood, spring being moist and warm.

You can learn the truth from the following facts. It is chiefly in spring and summer that men are attacked by dysenteries, and by hemorrhage from the nose, and they are then hottest and red. And in summer blood is still strong, and bile rises in the body and extends until autumn. In autumn blood becomes small in quantity, as autumn is opposed to its nature, while bile prevails in the body during the summer season and during autumn. You may learn this truth from the following facts. During this season men vomit bile without an emetic, and when they take purges the discharges are most bilious.

It is plain too from fevers and from the **complexions** of men. But in summer phlegm is at its weakest. For the season is opposed to its nature, being dry and warm. But in autumn blood becomes least in man, for autumn is dry and begins from this point to chill him. It is black bile which in autumn is greatest and strongest. When winter comes on, bile being chilled

sputum: Refers to mucus and coughed-up phlegm, both in Antiquity and today.

complexions: One of the most important concepts in Hippocratic-Galenic medicine, complexion refers to the combination of qualities and humors in every person, plant, animal, or food.

becomes small in quantity, and phlegm increases again because of the abundance of rain and the length of the nights. All these elements then are always comprised in the body of a man, but as the year goes round they become now greater and now less, each in turn and according to its nature. For just as every year participates in every element, the hot, the cold, the dry and the moist—none in fact of these elements would last for a moment without all the things that exist in this universe, but if one were to fail all would disappear, for by reason of the same necessity all things are constructed and nourished by one another—even so, if any of these congenital elements were to fail, the man could not live. In the year sometimes the winter is most powerful, sometimes the spring, sometimes the summer and sometimes the autumn. So too in man sometimes phlegm is powerful, sometimes blood, sometimes bile, first yellow, and then what is called black bile. The clearest proof is that if you will give the same man to drink the same drug four times in the year, he will vomit, you will find, the most phlegmatic matter in the winter, the moistest in the spring, the most bilious in the summer, and the blackest in the autumn....

XIII. Diseases which arise soon after their origin, and whose cause is clearly known, are those the history of which can be **foretold with the greatest certainty**. The patient himself must bring about a cure by combating the cause of the disease, for in this way will be removed that which caused the disease in the body.

XIV. Patients whose urine contains a deposit of sand or chalk suffer at first from tumors near the thick vein, with **suppuration**; then, since the tumors do not break quickly, from the pus there grow out pieces of chalk, which are pressed outside through the vein into the bladder with the urine. Those whose urine is merely blood-stained have suffered in the veins. When the urine is thick, and there are passed with it small pieces of flesh like hair, you must know that these symptoms result from the kidneys and arthritic complaints. When the urine is clear, but from time to time as it were bran appears in it, the patients suffer from psoriasis of the bladder.

XV. Most fevers come from bile. There are four sorts of them, apart from those that arise in distinctly separate pains. Their names are the continued, the **quotidian**, the **tertian**, and the **quartan**. Now what is called the continued fever comes from the most abundant and the purest bile, and its crises occur after the shortest interval. For since the body has no time to cool it wastes away rapidly, being warmed by the great heat. The quotidian next to the continued comes from the most abundant bile, and ceases quicker than any other, though it is longer than the continued, proportionately to

foretold with the greatest certainty: The author refers here to the art of prognosis, forecasting the progress of a disease and its expected outcome in recovery or death.

suppuration: The formation of pus.

quotidian: A fever that peaks and breaks once each day.

tertian: A fever that peaks and breaks every third day, measured inclusively (what we call every two days in modern counting).

quartan: A fever that peaks and breaks every fourth day, measured inclusively (what we call every three days in modern counting).

the lesser quantity of bile from which it comes; moreover the body has a breathing space, whereas in the continued there is no breathing space at all. The tertian is longer than the quotidian and is the result of less bile. The longer the breathing space enjoyed by the body in the case of the tertian than in the case of the quotidian, the longer this fever is than the quotidian. The quartans are in general similar, but they are more protracted than the tertians in so far as their portion is less of the bile that causes heat, while the intervals are greater in which the body cools.

It is from black bile that his excessive obstinacy arises. For black bile is the most viscous of the humors in the body, and that which sticks fast the longest. Hereby you will know that quartan fevers participate in the **atrabilious** element, because it is mostly in autumn that men are attacked by quartans, and between the ages of twenty-five and forty-five. This age is that which of all ages is most under the mastery of black bile, just as autumn is the season of all seasons which is most under its mastery. Such as are attacked by a quartan fever outside this period and this age you may be sure will not suffer from a long fever, unless the patient be the victim of another malady as well.

atrabilious: Relating to black (in Latin, *atra*) bile.

DOCUMENT 8:
Plato on the Nature of Disease: *Timaeus*[4]

Plato (ca. 428–348 BCE), in his dialogue *Timaeus*, explored human physiology and the causes of disease much like his contemporary Hippocrates and his students. Plato's dialogues are usually named after the main speaker who is conversing with Socrates. In this case it is one Timaeus of Locri, who is used to represent Plato's own ideas. Plato, like Hippocrates, considered disease to be the product of imbalance, but he focused on the four classical elements of earth, air, fire, and water rather than on the four humors of Hippocrates. He does mention humors like phlegm, but they are symptoms rather than foundational elements of his medical theory.

ℰ

Now everyone can see whence diseases arise. There are four natures out of which the body is compacted, earth and fire and water and air, and the unnatural excess or defect of these, or the change of any of them from its own natural place into another, or—since there are more kinds than one of fire and of the other elements—the assumption by any of these of a wrong kind, or any similar irregularity, produces disorders and diseases; for when any of them is produced or changed in a manner contrary to nature, the parts which were previously cool grow warm, and those which were dry become moist, and the light become heavy, and the heavy light; all sorts of changes occur. For, as we affirm, a thing can only remain the same with itself, whole and sound, when the same is added to it, or subtracted from it, in the same respect and in the same manner and in due proportion; and whatever comes or goes away in violation of these laws causes all manner of changes and infinite diseases and corruptions. Now there is a second class of structures which are also natural, and this affords a second opportunity of observing diseases to him who would understand them. For whereas marrow and bone and flesh and sinews are composed of the four elements, and the blood, though after another manner, is likewise formed out of them, most diseases originate in the way which I have described; but the worst of all owe their severity to the fact that the generation of these substances proceeds in a wrong order; they are then destroyed. For the natural order is that the flesh and sinews should be made of blood, the sinews out of the fibers to which they are akin, and the flesh out of the dots which are formed when the fibers are separated. And the glutinous and rich matter

---

4   Benjamin A. Jowett, translator, *The Dialogues of Plato*, Vol. III: *The Republic, Timaeus, Critias* (Macmillan and Company, 1892).

which comes away from the sinews and the flesh, not only glues the flesh to the bones, but nourishes and imparts growth to the bone which surrounds the marrow; and by reason of the solidity of the bones, that which filters through consists of the purest and smoothest and oiliest sort of triangles, dropping like dew from the bones and watering the marrow.

Now when each process takes place in this order, health commonly results; when in the opposite order, disease. For when the flesh becomes decomposed and sends back the wasting substance into the veins, then an over-supply of blood of diverse kinds, mingling with air in the veins, having variegated colors and bitter properties, as well as acid and saline qualities, contains all sorts of bile and serum and phlegm. For all things go the wrong way, and having become corrupted, first they taint the blood itself, and then ceasing to give nourishment to the body they are carried along the veins in all directions, no longer preserving the order of their natural courses, but at war with themselves, because they receive no good from one another, and are hostile to the abiding constitution of the body, which they corrupt and dissolve. The oldest part of the flesh which is corrupted, being hard to decompose, from long burning grows black, and from being everywhere corroded becomes bitter, and is injurious to every part of the body which is still uncorrupted. Sometimes, when the bitter element is refined away, the black part assumes an acidity which takes the place of the bitterness; at other times the bitterness being tinged with blood has a redder color; and this, when mixed with black, takes the hue of grass; and again, an auburn color mingles with the bitter matter when new flesh is decomposed by the fire which surrounds the internal flame—to all which symptoms some physician perhaps, or rather some philosopher, who had the power of seeing in many dissimilar things one nature deserving of a name, has assigned the common name of bile. But the other kinds of bile are variously distinguished by their colors. As for serum, that sort which is the watery part of blood is innocent, but that which is a secretion of black and acid bile is malignant when mingled by the power of heat with any salt substance, and is then called acid phlegm.

DOCUMENT 9:

Thucydides and the Plague of Athens, 430 BCE[5]

Thucydides (460–395 BCE) described a plague that struck Athens in 430 BCE (not bubonic plague, but possibly typhus or typhoid) during their war with Sparta. In this passage from his *History of the Peloponnesian War*, written around 20 years after the plague, in 410 BCE, Thucydides describes the disease's progress, symptoms, and effects, but does not explore its cause.

e

In the first days of summer the Spartans and their allies, with two-thirds of their forces as before, invaded Attica, under the command of Archidamus, son of Zeuxidamus, king of Sparta, and sat down and laid waste the country. Not many days after their arrival in Attica the plague first began to show itself among the Athenians. It was said that it had broken out in many places previously in the neighborhood of Lemnos and elsewhere; but a pestilence of such extent and mortality was nowhere remembered. Neither were the physicians at first of any service, ignorant as they were of the proper way to treat it, but they died themselves the most thickly, as they visited the sick most often; nor did any human art succeed any better. Supplications in the temples, divinations, and so forth were found equally futile, till the overwhelming nature of the disaster at last put a stop to them altogether.

It first began, it is said, in the parts of Ethiopia above Egypt, and thence descended into Egypt and Libya and into most of the King's country. Suddenly falling upon Athens, it first attacked the population in Piraeus—which was the occasion of their saying that the Peloponnesians had poisoned the reservoirs, there being as yet no wells there—and afterwards appeared in the upper city, when the deaths became much more frequent. All speculation as to its origin and its causes, if causes can be found adequate to produce so great a disturbance, I leave to other writers, whether lay or professional; for myself, I shall simply set down its nature, and explain the symptoms by which perhaps it may be recognized by the student, if it should ever break out again. This I can the better do, as I had the disease myself, and watched its operation in the case of others.

That year then is admitted to have been otherwise unprecedentedly free from sickness; and such few cases as occurred all determined in this. As a rule, however, there was no ostensible cause; but people in good health were all of a sudden attacked by violent heats in the head, and redness and

---

5   Thucydides, *History of the Peloponnesian War*, translated by Richard Crawley (J.M. Dent & Sons, 1914), II.47–54.

inflammation in the eyes, the inward parts, such as the throat or tongue, becoming bloody and emitting an unnatural and fetid breath. These symptoms were followed by sneezing and hoarseness, after which the pain soon reached the chest, and produced a hard cough. When it fixed in the stomach, it upset it; and discharges of bile of every kind named by physicians ensued, accompanied by very great distress. In most cases also an ineffectual retching followed, producing violent spasms, which in some cases ceased soon after, in others much later. Externally the body was not very hot to the touch, nor pale in its appearance, but reddish, livid, and breaking out into small pustules and ulcers. But internally it burned so that the patient could not bear to have on him clothing or linen even of the very lightest description; or indeed to be otherwise than stark naked. What they would have liked best would have been to throw themselves into cold water; as indeed was done by some of the neglected sick, who plunged into the rain tanks in their agonies of unquenchable thirst; though it made no difference whether they drank little or much. Besides this, the miserable feeling of not being able to rest or sleep never ceased to torment them. The body meanwhile did not waste away so long as the distemper was at its height, but held out to a marvel against its ravages; so that when they succumbed, as in most cases, on the seventh or eighth day to the internal inflammation, they had still some strength in them. But if they passed this stage, and the disease descended further into the bowels, inducing a violent ulceration there accompanied by severe diarrhœa, this brought on a weakness which was generally fatal. For the disorder first settled in the head, ran its course from thence through the whole of the body, and, even where it did not prove mortal, it still left its mark on the extremities; for it settled in the privy parts, the fingers and the toes, and many escaped with the loss of these, some too with that of their eyes. Others again were seized with an entire loss of memory on their first recovery, and did not know either themselves or their friends.

But while the nature of the distemper was such as to baffle all description, and its attacks almost too grievous for human nature to endure, it was still in the following circumstance that its difference from all ordinary disorders was most clearly shown. All the birds and beasts that prey upon human bodies, either abstained from touching them (though there were many lying unburied), or died after tasting them. In proof of this, it was noticed that birds of this kind actually disappeared; they were not about the bodies, or indeed to be seen at all. But of course the effects which I have mentioned could best be studied in a domestic animal like the dog.

Such then, if we pass over the varieties of particular cases which were many and peculiar, were the general features of the distemper. Meanwhile the town enjoyed an immunity from all the ordinary disorders; or if any case occurred, it ended in this. Some died in neglect, others in the midst of every attention. No remedy was found that could be used as a specific; for what did good in one case, did harm in another. Strong and weak constitutions proved equally incapable of resistance, all alike being swept away, although dieted with the utmost precaution. By far the most terrible feature in the malady was the dejection which ensued when any one felt himself sickening, for the despair into which they instantly fell took away their power of resistance, and left them a much easier prey to the disorder; besides which, there was the awful spectacle of men dying like sheep, through having caught the infection in nursing each other. This caused the greatest mortality. On the one hand, if they were afraid to visit each other, they perished from neglect; indeed many houses were emptied of their inmates for want of a nurse: on the other, if they ventured to do so, death was the consequence. This was especially the case with such as made any pretensions to goodness: honour made them unsparing of themselves in their attendance in their friends' houses, where even the members of the family were at last worn out by the moans of the dying, and succumbed to the force of the disaster. Yet it was with those who had recovered from the disease that the sick and the dying found most compassion. These knew what it was from experience, and had now no fear for themselves; for the same man was never attacked twice—never at least fatally. And such persons not only received the congratulations of others, but themselves also, in the elation of the moment, half entertained the vain hope that they were for the future safe from any disease whatsoever.

An aggravation of the existing calamity was the influx from the country into the city, and this was especially felt by the new arrivals. As there were no houses to receive them, they had to be lodged at the hot season of the year in stifling cabins, where the mortality raged without restraint. The bodies of dying men lay one upon another, and half-dead creatures reeled about the streets and gathered round all the fountains in their longing for water. The sacred places also in which they had quartered themselves were full of corpses of persons that had died there, just as they were; for as the disaster passed all bounds, men, not knowing what was to become of them, became utterly careless of everything, whether sacred or profane. All the burial rites before in use were entirely upset, and they buried the bodies as best they could. Many from want of the proper appliances, through so many of their friends having died already, had recourse to the most shameless sepultures: sometimes getting the start of those who had raised a pile, they threw their own dead body upon the stranger's pyre and ignited it; sometimes they tossed the corpse which they were carrying on the top of another that was burning, and so went off.

Nor was this the only form of lawless extravagance which owed its origin to the plague. Men now coolly ventured on what they had formerly done in a corner, and not just as they pleased, seeing the rapid transitions produced by persons in prosperity suddenly dying and those who before had nothing succeeding to their property. So they resolved to spend quickly and enjoy themselves, regarding their lives and riches as alike things of a day. Perseverance in what men called honour was popular with none, it was so uncertain whether they would be spared to attain the object; but it was settled that present enjoyment, and all that contributed to it, was both honourable and useful. Fear of gods or law of man there was none to restrain them. As for the first, they judged it to be just the same whether they worshipped them or not, as they saw all alike perishing; and for the last, no one expected to live to be brought to trial for his offences, but each felt that a far severer sentence had been already passed upon them all and hung ever over their heads, and before this fell it was only reasonable to enjoy life a little.

Such was the nature of the calamity, and heavily did it weigh on the Athenians; death raging within the city and devastation without.

DOCUMENT 10:

Hippocratic Corpus, *Aphorisms*[6]

One of the most important Hippocratic teaching texts is the *Aphorisms*, a collection of brief statements about medicine, some straightforward, but many enigmatic in nature. These were probably compiled and written down by Hippocrates' followers in the fourth century BCE. Although the *Aphorisms* lack the rational organization and clear medical details of treatises like *Nature of Man* (Document 7, pp. 29–32) or *On the Sacred Disease*, it nonetheless became central to Hellenistic and Roman medicine, and was translated multiple times into Latin, Arabic, Hebrew, and European vernaculars during the Middle Ages. Students of medicine in European universities wrote commentaries on the *Aphorisms* as a valid source of medical information well beyond the Middle Ages, even into the eighteenth century.

ॐ

1. Life is short, and Art long; the **crisis** fleeting; experience perilous, and decision difficult. The physician must not only be prepared to do what is right himself, but also to make the patient, the attendants, and externals cooperate.

2. In disorders of the bowels and vomitings, occurring spontaneously, if the matters purged be such as ought to be purged, they do good, and are well borne; but if not, the contrary. And so **artificial evacuations**, if they consist of such matters as should be evacuated, do good, and are well borne; but if not, the contrary. One, then, ought to look to the **country, the season, the age**, and the diseases in which they are proper or not.

3. In athletes, stoutness, if carried to its utmost limit, is dangerous, for they cannot remain in the same state nor be stationary; and since, then, they can neither remain stationary nor improve, it only remains for them to get worse; for these reasons the stoutness should be reduced without delay, that the body may again have a commencement of reparation. Neither should the evacuations, in their case, be carried to an extreme, for this also is dangerous, but only to such a point as the person's constitution can endure. In like manner, medicinal evacuations, if carried to an extreme, are dangerous; and again, a restorative course, if in the extreme, is dangerous.

4. A slender restricted diet is always dangerous in chronic diseases, and also in acute diseases, where it is not requisite. And again, a diet brought

crisis: The turning point of a disease, either for better or worse. The term especially was used to refer to the point at which a patient's fever grew worst, broke, and led to recovery or death.

artificial evacuations: Purgations by vomiting, urine, or stool caused by a medicine, enema, or other artificial method.

country, the season, the age: This idea of understanding the patient's country and environment is explored in greater detail in the Hippocratic work *Airs, Waters, Places* in Document 11.

6   Francis Adams, *The Genuine Works of Hippocrates* (Dover, 1868).

to the extreme point of attenuation is dangerous; and repletion, when in the extreme, is also dangerous.

5. In a restricted diet, patients who transgress are thereby more hurt (than in any other?); for every such transgression, whatever it may be, is followed by greater consequences than in a diet somewhat more generous. On this account, a very slender, regulated, and restricted diet is dangerous to persons in health, because they bear transgressions of it more difficultly. For this reason, a slender and restricted diet is generally more dangerous than one a little more liberal.

6. For extreme diseases, extreme methods of cure, as to restriction, are most suitable.

7. When the disease is very acute, it is attended with extremely severe symptoms in its first stage; and therefore an extremely attenuating diet must be used. When this is not the case, but it is allowable to give a more generous diet, we may depart as far from the severity of **regimen** as the disease, by its mildness, is removed from the extreme.

8. When the disease is at its height, it will then be necessary to use the most slender diet.

9. We must form a particular judgment of the patient, whether he will support the diet until the acme of the disease, and whether he will sink previously and not support the diet, or the disease will give way previously, and become less acute.

10. In those cases, then, which attain their acme speedily, a restricted diet should be enjoined at first; but in those cases which reach their acme later, we must retrench at that period or a little before it; but previously we must allow a more generous diet to support the patient.

11. We must retrench during **paroxysms**, for to exhibit food would be injurious. And in all diseases having periodical paroxysms, we must restrict during the paroxysms.

12. The exacerbations and remissions will be indicated by the diseases, the seasons of the year, the reciprocation of the periods, whether they occur every day, every alternate day, or after a longer period, and by the supervening symptoms; as, for example, in **pleuritic** cases, expectoration, if it occur at the commencement, shortens the attack, but if it appear later, it prolongs the same; and in the same manner the urine, and **alvine** discharges, and sweats, according as they appear along with favorable or unfavorable symptoms, indicate diseases of a short or long duration.

13. Old persons endure fasting most easily; next, adults; young persons not nearly so well; and most especially infants, and of them such as are of a particularly lively spirit.

14. Growing bodies have the most innate heat; they therefore require the most food, for otherwise their bodies are wasted. In old persons the heat

regimen: A schedule of diet, rest, and physical activity prescribed by a physician, especially one trained in Hippocratic humoral theory.

paroxysms: Violent attacks of any medical symptoms, but here apparently nausea and fever.

pleuritic: Suffering from pleurisy, the painful collection of fluids or inflammation of the membranes around the lungs, called *pleurae* in Latin.

alvine: Relating to the belly or intestines.

is feeble, and therefore they require little fuel, as it were, to the flame, for it would be extinguished by much. On this account, also, fevers in old persons are not equally acute, because their bodies are cold.

15. In winter and spring the bowels are naturally the hottest, and the sleep most prolonged; at these seasons, then, the most sustenance is to be administered; for as the belly has then most innate heat, it stands in need of most food. The well-known facts with regard to young persons and the athletes prove this.

16. A humid regimen is befitting in all febrile diseases, and particularly in children, and others accustomed to live on such a diet.

17. We must consider, also, in which cases food is to be given once or twice a day, and in greater or smaller quantities, and at intervals. Something must be conceded to habit, to season, to country, and to age.

18. Invalids bear food worst during summer and autumn, most easily in winter, and next in spring.

19. Neither give nor enjoin anything to persons during periodical paroxysms, but abstract from the accustomed allowance before the crisis.

20. When things are at the crisis, or when they have just passed it, neither move the bowels, nor make any innovation in the treatment, either as regards **purgatives** or any other such stimulants, but let things alone.

21. Those things which require to be evacuated should be evacuated, wherever they most tend, by the proper outlets.

22. We must purge and move such humors as are **concocted**, not such as are **unconcocted**, unless they are struggling to get out, which is mostly not the case.

23. The evacuations are to be judged of not by their quantity, but whether they be such as they should be, and how they are borne. And when proper to carry the evacuation to *deliquium animi*, this also should be done, provided the patient can support it.

24. Use purgative medicines sparingly in acute diseases, and at the commencement, and not without proper circumspection.

25. If the matters which are purged be such as should be purged, the evacuation is beneficial, and easily borne; but, not withstanding, if otherwise, with difficulty.

purgatives: A medicine or medical action designed to remove bad or excess humors from the body. These usually took the form of bloodletting or cupping, as well as drugs that caused vomiting, emetics for increased urination, or enemas. Women could also be prescribed emmenagogues, drugs that caused or increased menstruation.

concocted ... unconcocted: Coction is the "cooking" of humors within the body, sometimes beneficial (as with the growth of children) and sometimes harmful (as with the corruption of humors leading to dangerous diseases).

deliquium animi: Latin for a "failure of the spirit," i.e., fainting.

DOCUMENT 11:

Hippocratic Corpus, *Airs, Waters, Places*[7]

For a Hippocratic physician to diagnose a disease properly and determine the correct form of treatment, he needed to understand fully the patient's native environment. The author of *Airs, Waters, Places* (later fifth century BCE), assumes that a doctor travels and will come "into a city to which he is a stranger." He can gain new patients and income by impressing people with his knowledge of their own landscape and environment. The author especially recognized the importance of water quality, for without modern water treatment, every region and community had its own varieties of water, differing in flavor, salinity, microbes, minerals, and healthfulness. There were different kinds of good water and different kinds of bad, all of which a good physician needed to understand before he could correctly diagnose a disease and determine a suitable remedy for the patient.[8]

ç

PART 1. Whoever wishes to investigate medicine properly, should proceed thus: in the first place to consider the seasons of the year, and what effects each of them produces for they are not at all alike, but differ much from themselves in regard to their changes. Then the winds, the hot and the cold, especially such as are common to all countries, and then such as are peculiar to each locality. We must also consider the qualities of the waters, for as they differ from one another in taste and weight, so also do they differ much in their qualities. In the same manner, when one comes into a city to which he is a stranger, he ought to consider its situation, how it lies as to the winds and the rising of the sun; for its influence is not the same whether it lies to the north or the south, to the rising or to the setting sun. These things one ought to consider most attentively, and concerning the waters which the inhabitants use, whether they be marshy and soft, or hard, and running from elevated and rocky situations, and then if salty and unfit for cooking; and the ground, whether it be naked and deficient in water, or wooded and well watered, and whether it lies in a hollow, confined situation, or is elevated and cold; and the mode in which the inhabitants live, and what are their pursuits, whether they are fond of drinking and eating to excess, and given to indolence, or are fond of exercise and labor, and not given to excess in eating and drinking.

---

7   Francis Adams, *The Genuine Works of Hippocrates* (Dover, 1868).

8   Jacques Jouanna, "Water, Health and Disease in the Hippocratic Treatise *Airs, Waters, Places*," in *Greek Medicine from Hippocrates to Galen: Selected Papers*, edited by Philip van der Eijk and translated by Neil Allies (Brill, 2012), 155–72.

PART 2. From these things he must proceed to investigate everything else. For if one knows all these things well, or at least the greater part of them, he cannot miss knowing, when he comes into a strange city, either the diseases peculiar to the place, or the particular nature of common diseases, so that he will not be in doubt as to the treatment of the diseases, or commit mistakes, as is likely to be the case provided one had not previously considered these matters. And in particular, as the season and the year advances, he can tell what epidemic diseases will attack the city, either in summer or in winter, and what each individual will be in danger of experiencing from the change of regimen. For knowing the changes of the seasons, the risings and settings of the stars, how each of them takes place, he will be able to know beforehand what sort of a year is going to ensue. Having made these investigations, and knowing beforehand the seasons, such a one must be acquainted with each particular, and must succeed in the preservation of health, and be by no means unsuccessful in the practice of his art. And if it shall be thought that these things belong rather to meteorology, it will be admitted, on second thoughts, that astronomy contributes not a little, but a very great deal, indeed, to medicine. For with the seasons the digestive organs of men undergo a change.

PART 3. But how of the aforementioned things should be investigated and explained, I will now declare in a clear manner. A city that is exposed to hot winds (these are between the wintry rising, and the wintry setting of the sun), and to which these are peculiar, but which is sheltered from the north winds; in such a city the waters will be plenteous and salty, and as they run from an elevated source, they are necessarily hot in summer, and cold in winter; the heads of the inhabitants are of a humid and **pituitous** constitution, and their bellies subject to frequent disorders, owing to the phlegm running down from the head; the forms of their bodies, for the most part, are rather flabby; they do not eat nor drink much; drinking wine in particular, and more especially if carried to intoxication, is oppressive to them; and the following diseases are peculiar to the district: in the first place, the women are sickly and subject to excessive menstruation; then many are unfruitful from disease, and not from nature, and they have frequent miscarriages; infants are subject to attacks of convulsions and asthma, which they consider to be connected with infancy, and hold to be a **sacred disease**. The men are subject to attacks of dysentery, diarrhea, **hepialus**, chronic fevers in winter, of **epinyctis**, frequently, and of hemorrhoids about the anus. **Pleurisies**, **peripneumonies**, ardent fevers, and whatever diseases are reckoned **acute**, do not often occur, for such diseases are not apt to prevail where the bowels are loose. **Ophthalmies** occur of a humid character, but not of a serious nature, and of short duration, unless they attack epidemically from the change of

pituitous: Full of mucus or phlegm.

sacred disease: Epilepsy was known as the "sacred disease" because many ancient people thought it was caused by a god or a spirit, an idea Hippocrates denies in his revolutionary work on epilepsy, *On the Sacred Disease*.

hepialus: A type of intermittent fever common in warm climates or seasons. It is here distinguished from the chronic fevers in cold seasons.

epinyctis: Sores on the eyelid or any kind of pustule.

Pleurisies: The painful collection of fluids or inflammation of the membranes around the lungs, called *pleurae*.

peripneumonies: An older term for pneumonia, perhaps a serious or recurrent pneumonic condition.

acute: Both ancient and modern physicians frequently classify diseases as acute (coming on suddenly and sharply) or chronic (long-lasting and developing slowly).

Ophthalmies: A severe inflammation of the eye, such as from conjunctivitis (pink eye).

the seasons. And when they pass their fiftieth year, defluxions supervening from the brain,[9] render them paralytic when exposed suddenly to strokes of the sun, or to cold. These diseases are endemic to them, and, moreover, if any epidemic disease connected with the change of the seasons, prevail, they are also liable to it.

PART 4. But the following is the condition of cities which have the opposite exposure, namely, to cold winds, between the summer settings and the summer risings of the sun, and to which these winds are peculiar, and which are sheltered from the south and the hot breezes. In the first place the waters are, for the most part, hard cold. The men must necessarily be well braced and slender, and they must have the discharges downwards of the alimentary canal hard, and of difficult evacuation, while those upwards are more fluid, and rather **bilious than pituitous**. Their heads are sound and hard, and they are liable to burstings (of vessels?) for the most part. The diseases which prevail epidemically with them, are pleurisies, and those which are called acute diseases. This must be the case when the bowels are bound; and from any causes, many become affected with suppurations in the lungs, the cause of which is the tension of the body, and hardness of the bowels; for their dryness and the coldness of the water dispose them to ruptures. Such constitutions must be given to excess of eating, but not of drinking; for it is not possible to be gourmands and drunkards at the same time. Ophthalmies, too, at length supervene; these being of a hard and violent nature, and soon ending in rupture of the eyes; persons under thirty years of age are liable to severe bleedings at the nose in summer; attacks of epilepsy are rare but severe. Such people are likely to be rather long-lived; their ulcers are not attended with serious discharges, nor of a malignant character; in disposition they are rather ferocious than gentle. The diseases I have mentioned are peculiar to the men, and besides they are liable to any common complaint which may be prevailing from the changes of the seasons. But the women, in the first place, are of a hard constitution, from the waters being hard, indigestible, and cold; and their menstrual discharges are not regular, but in small quantity, and painful. Then they have difficult **parturition**, but are not very subject to **abortions**. And when they do bring forth children, they are unable to nurse them; for the hardness and indigestible nature of the water puts away their milk. **Phthisis** frequently supervenes after childbirth, for the efforts of it frequently bring on ruptures and strains. Children while still little are subject to dropsies in the testicle, which disappear as they grow older; in

bilious than pituitous: Meaning their humors tend more toward bile than phlegm.

parturition: The act of giving birth.

abortion: In premodern and early modern texts, the term was used both for intentional abortion of the fetus and unintentional miscarriages. You must read the text carefully to determine which is meant.

Phthisis: Pulmonary tuberculosis.

9   It was assumed that the brain could produce humors which, when in excess, could flow down ("defluxions") into the body and disturb the humoral balance. This concept is also found among the ancient Egyptians, who considered the brain primarily as a source of mucus rather than an organ of thought.

such a town they are late in attaining manhood. It is, as I have now stated, with regard to hot and cold winds and cities thus exposed.

PART 5. Cities that are exposed to winds between the summer and the winter risings of the sun, and those the opposite to them, have the following characters: Those which lie to the rising of the sun are all likely to be more healthy than such as are turned to the North, or those exposed to the hot winds, even if there should not be a furlong between them. In the first place, both the heat and cold are more moderate. Then such waters as flow to the rising sun, must necessarily be clear, fragrant, soft, and delightful to drink, in such a city. For the sun in rising and shining upon them purifies them, by dispelling the vapors which generally prevail in the morning. The persons of the inhabitants are, for the most part, well colored and blooming, unless some disease counteract. The inhabitants have clear voices, and in temper and intellect are superior to those which are exposed to the north, and all the productions of the country in like manner are better. A city so situated resembles the spring as to moderation between heat and cold, and the diseases are few in number, and of a feeble kind, and bear a resemblance to the diseases which prevail in regions exposed to hot winds. The women there are very prolific, and have easy deliveries. Thus it is with regard to them.

PART 6. But such cities as lie to the west, and which are sheltered from winds blowing from the east, and which the hot winds and the cold winds of the north scarcely touch, must necessarily be in a very unhealthy situation: in the first place the waters are not clear, the cause of which is, because the mist prevails commonly in the morning, and it is mixed up with the water and destroys its clearness, for the sun does not shine upon the water until he be considerably raised above the horizon. And in summer, cold breezes from the east blow and dews fall; and in the latter part of the day the setting sun particularly scorches the inhabitants, and therefore they are pale and enfeebled, and are partly subject to all the aforesaid diseases, but no one is peculiar to them. Their voices are rough and hoarse owing to the state of the air, which in such a situation is generally impure and unwholesome, for they have not the northern winds to purify it; and these winds they have are of a very humid character, such being the nature of the evening breezes. Such a situation of a city bears a great resemblance to autumn as regards the changes of the day, inasmuch as the difference between morning and evening is great. So it is with regard to the winds that are conducive to health, or the contrary.

DOCUMENT 12:

Case Histories from the Hippocratic *Epidemics*[10]

The Hippocratic text *Epidemics* is organized into seven books written over a period of many decades (later fifth and early fourth centuries BCE), possibly by the real Hippocrates and then by some of his followers. The authors provide detailed descriptions of the symptoms and outcome (usually death) of patients suffering from some sort of feverish epidemic disease. The opening paragraph lays out the theoretical foundations for the observations made in the individual cases and represents ideas very similar to those found in the Hippocratic *Airs, Waters, Places* (Document 11).

⸱⸱

With regard to diseases, the circumstances from which we form a judgment of them are, by attending to the general nature of all, and the peculiar nature of each individual, to the disease, the patient, and the applications, to the person who applies them, as that makes a difference for better or for worse, to the whole constitution of the season, and particularly to the **state of the heavens**, and the **nature of each country**; to the patient's habits, regimen, and pursuits; to his conversation, manners, taciturnity, thoughts, sleep, or absence of sleep, and sometimes his dreams, what and when they occur; to his picking and scratching; to his tears; to the alvine discharges, urine, sputa, and vomitings; and to the **changes of diseases from the one into the other**; to the deposits, whether of a deadly or critical character; to the sweat, coldness, rigor, cough, sneezing, hiccup, respiration, eructation, flatulence, whether passed silently or with a noise; to hemorrhages and hemorrhoids; from these, and their consequences, we must form a judgment....

Case 9. Criton, in Thasus, while still on foot, and going about, was seized with a violent pain in the great toe; he took to bed the same day, had rigors and nausea, recovered his heat slightly, at night was delirious. On the second, swelling of the whole foot, and about the ankle *erythema*, with distention, and small *bullae*; acute fever; he became furiously deranged; alvine discharges bilious, unmixed, and rather frequent. He died on the second day from the commencement.

Case 10. The Clazomenian who was lodged by the Well of Phrynichides was seized with fever. He had pain in the head, neck, and loins from the beginning, and immediately afterwards deafness; tongue dry. On the fourth,

---

state of the heavens: Astrology was a regular part of medicine in the ancient and medieval worlds, and generally not associated with magic or superstition as it is today.

nature of each country: See Document 11, pp. 42–45, for the Hippocratic *Airs, Waters, Places*, which teaches the physician how to judge "the nature of each country" in medical terms.

changes of diseases from the one into the other: Ancient physicians did not understand a "disease" to be caused by a unique pathogen or a single physical condition, but rather as one or more definable symptoms, which could transform into another "disease" as the symptoms changed (even if we now understand that all those symptoms had a single cause).

erythema: Any reddening of the skin.

bullae: Blisters or pustules.

---

10 *The Genuine Works of Hippocrates*, translated by Francis Adams (The Sydenham Society, 1849).

towards night, he became delirious. On the fifth, in an uneasy state. On the sixth, all the symptoms exacerbated. About the eleventh a slight remission; from the commencement to the fourteenth day the alvine discharges thin, copious, and of the color of water, but were well supported; the bowels then became constipated. Urine throughout thin, and well colored, and had many substances scattered through it, but no sediment. About the sixteenth, urine somewhat thicker, which had a slight sediment; somewhat better, and more collected. On the seventeenth, urine again thin; swellings about both his ears, with pain; no sleep, some incoherence; legs painfully affected. On the twentieth, free of fever, had a crisis, no sweat, perfectly collected. About the twenty-seventh, violent pain of the right hip; it speedily went off. The swellings about the ears subsided, and did not suppurate, but were painful. About the thirty-first, a diarrhea attended with a copious discharge of watery matter, and symptoms of dysentery; passed thick urine; swellings about the ears gone. About the fortieth day, had pain in the right eye, sight dull. It went away.

Case 11. The wife of Dromeades having been delivered of a female child, and all other matters going on properly, on the second day after was seized with rigor and acute fever. Began to have pain about the **hypochondrium** on the first day; had nausea and incoherence, and for some hours afterwards had no sleep; respiration rare, large, and suddenly interrupted. On the day following that on which she had the rigor, alvine discharges proper; **urine** thick, white, muddy, like urine which has been shaken after standing for some time, until the sediment had fallen to the bottom; it had no sediment; she did not sleep during the night. On the third day, about noon, had a rigor, acute fever; urine the same; pain of the hypochondria, nausea, an uncomfortable night, no sleep; a coldish sweat all over, but heat quickly restored. On the fourth, slight alleviation of the symptoms about the hypochondria; heaviness of the head, with pain; somewhat comatose; slight *epistaxis*, tongue dry, thirst, urine thin and oily; slept a little, upon awaking was somewhat comatose; slight coldness, slept during the night, was delirious. On the morning of the sixth had a rigor, but soon recovered her heat, sweated all over; extremities cold, was delirious, respiration rare and large. Shortly afterwards spasms from the head began, and she immediately expired.

Case 12. A man, in a heated state, took supper, and drank more than enough; he vomited the whole during the night; acute fever, pain of the right hypochondrium, a softish inflammation from the inner part; passed an uncomfortable night; urine at the commencement thick, red, but when allowed to stand, had no sediment, tongue dry, and not very thirsty. On the fourth, acute fever, pains all over. On the fifth, urine smooth, oily, and

hypochondrium: The upper part of the abdomen, stretching over the lower ribs.

urine: This close analysis of urine for the purpose of medical diagnosis or prognosis came to be called uroscopy or urinalysis, and a central feature of medieval medicine.

epistaxis: A nosebleed.

copious; acute fever. On the sixth, in the evening, very incoherent, no sleep during the night. On the seventh, all the symptoms exacerbated; urine of the same characters; much talking, and he could not contain himself; the bowels being stimulated, passed a water discharge with *lumbrici*: night equally painful. On the morning had a rigor; acute fever, hot sweat, appeared to be free of fever; did not sleep long; after the sleep a chill, **ptyalism**; in the evening, a great incoherence; after a little, vomited a small quantity of dark bilious matters. On the ninth, coldness, much delirium, did not sleep. On the tenth, pains in the limbs, all the symptoms exacerbated; he was delirious. On the eleventh, he died....

Case 14. Melidia, who lodged near the Temple of Juno, began to feel a violent pain of the head, neck, and chest. She was straightway seized with acute fever; a slight appearance of the menses; continued pains of all these parts. On the sixth, was affected with coma, nausea, and rigor; redness about the cheeks; slight delirium. On the seventh, had a sweat; the fever intermitted, the pains remained. A relapse; little sleep; urine throughout of a good color, but thin; the alvine evacuations were thin, bilious, acrid, very scanty, black, and fetid; a white smooth sediment in the urine; had a sweat, and experienced a **perfect crisis** on the eleventh day.

lumbrici: Intestinal parasites or worms.

ptyalism: Excessive salivation.

perfect crisis: The crisis is the turning point of a disease, either for better or worse. Here, a perfect crisis is when the fever and other symptoms reach a peak and clear up entirely.

Hippocrates and his rationalized medicine can, at times, overshadow a complete understanding of classical medicine. Most ancient people living within ancient Greek or Roman cultures turned as much (if not more) to priests and gods as to physicians and medical theory to help with sickness and injury. Nearly every god of the ancient world could heal his or her followers, and some were directly associated with medicine. For the Greeks, Apollo was associated with both healing and plagues (see Document 4, pp. 19–20), as was Artemis, goddess of the hunt. But one god in particular came to be associated directly with the practice of medicine around the Mediterranean: Asclepius (Greek *Asklepios*, Latin *Aesculapius*). According to classical myths, Asclepius was a demi-god, the son of Apollo and a mortal woman. The wise centaur Chiron raised him and taught him medicine.

The Greek lyric poet Pindar (ca. 552–443 BCE) records one of the earliest versions of this story in Document 14. But not long after Pindar, Hippocrates himself may also have shown his devotion to Asclepius in one of the most famous documents in ancient medicine, the Hippocratic *Oath* (Document 13). The oath is still said (in modernized and secularized forms) at medical schools around the world. There is vigorous debate among historians of medicine about the author and date of the *Oath*, with arguments ranging from Hippocrates himself in the fifth century BCE to early Christians in the first or second century CE. If it is a genuinely early document, then it places Hippocratic medicine in a religious context: his students and followers had to swear before the healing gods Apollo, Asclepius, Hygieia, and Panacea to protect the secrets and reputation of medicine as taught and practiced in the "school" of Hippocrates.

The Greek gods of medicine Apollo, Chiron, and Asclepius were adopted by the Romans along with Greek medical theory and practice. They are portrayed together in a first-century CE fresco from the Roman city of Pompeii, as the founders and divine protectors of medicine. A Roman author, Hyginus (d. 17 CE), elaborated in his *Fables* on the specific medical contributions of these three "founders" of medicine: "Chiron the centaur, son of Saturn, first established the art of medical surgery using herbs. Apollo first practiced the art of medicine for eyes. In the third place Asclepius, son of Apollo, discovered the art of clinical medicine."[11] Hyginus used the Greek word *clinicen* to refer to the rational, formalized medicine of Asclepius and (implicitly) Hippocrates. This provides further evidence that the Romans

---

11   *Hygini Fabulae* no. 274, edited by M. Schmidt (Jena, 1872), 149–50. Original translation by the editor of this volume.

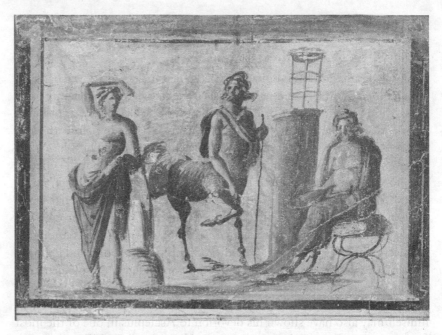

Apollo, Chiron, and Asclepius, from a first-century CE fresco in Pompeii

considered learned medicine to be primarily a Greek affair. According to legend, Asclepius had five divine daughters, each associated with a branch of health or healing: Hygieia, Panacea ("All-Heal"), Aceso, Iaso, and Aglaea. The first daughter lives on in our word "hygiene." Zeus, the father of the gods, killed Asclepius with a lightning bolt when he overstepped the bounds of human medicine, raising a man from the dead and accepting a payment for it. Asclepius may have been a real healer, and some ancient and medieval authors treat him not as a god, but as a wise human being such as Celsus in the first century CE (Document 15) and St. Isidore of Seville in the seventh century (Document 36, pp. 109–10). Celsus claims that the primitive Greeks thought Asclepius was a god because he practiced medicine at a time when the art was scarcely known.

Temples dedicated to Asclepius, called *asklepieia* (singular *asklepieion*), were established throughout the Greco-Roman world at least since the fifth century BCE. Hippocrates himself may have trained at the *asklepieion* on his home island of Kos. Both priests and physicians served at these temples, where the sick and injured came to seek healing. Patients who were healed, or were hoping for healing, left offerings called votives which often depicted the part of the body where they were suffering, like the leg-shaped votive left by one Tyche at a healing temple in the second century CE (Document 16). Thousands of these anatomical votives survive from the ancient world, and represent every major body part (head, hands, breasts, genitals, etc.) and internal organ (bladder, intestines, and uterus). They give us an indication of the popular understanding of internal anatomy in the ancient world.

According to Roman tradition, the cult of Asclepius was introduced to Rome after 295 BCE when a plague devastated the city, and the desperate Romans, rarely ones to rely on foreign gods during their early Republican period, decided to appeal to this Greek god of healing. After a temple to Asclepius was built on an island in the Tiber River, the plague disappeared. This assured the popularity and permanent presence of Asclepius among the Roman gods. John Scarborough goes so far as to call "The introduction of Asclepius ... the first event of 'medical history' at Rome."[12] Asclepius was not a typical god of healing, but a specialized god specifically of medicine and doctors. His divine power could help physicians practice medicine—and their patients heal—more efficiently.

Later Roman devotion to Asclepius is especially evident in the writings of Aelius Aristides (117–181 CE), perhaps the most famous invalid of classical Rome. Although Aristides was a famous orator in his own day, who made many speaking tours throughout the Empire, and the author of many surviving set speeches, he is now best known for recording his illnesses and their medical-religious treatments. He seems to have been genuinely ill in a variety of ways, but also a hypochondriac and eager for medical and religious attention. We know much about his ailments and cures because he recorded many of his visits between 145 and 170 CE to *asklepieia* and other medical sanctuaries in his *Sacred Tales*. The passages in Document 17 come from Aristides' record of one of his most serious episodes of illness: in the winter of the year 166, he suffered from chronic abdominal pain and vomiting. Dreams sent by Asclepius indicated that Aristides should abstain from bathing, and instead employ bleeding, enemas, and strange diets.

One of the most important cultural developments in the Hellenistic period was the mixing of classical Greek culture and religion with those of the non-Greek peoples conquered by Alexander the Great. A clear example of this mixing, called "syncretism" by anthropologists, can be seen in one of the Oxyrhyncus Papyri, a large collection of Greek and Latin texts written primarily on papyrus, between the first and sixth centuries CE in Roman Egypt. The passage in Document 18 is a translation of a Greek account written in the second century CE about the god "Imouthes," the Greek interpretation of Imhotep, the Egyptian patron of physicians and a healer of diseases. The entire description, however, is dependent on ideas about the Greek god Asclepius, who came to sick people in dreams, as seen in the account of Aelius Aristides (Document 17).

---

12   John Scarborough, *Roman Medicine* (Thames and Hudson, 1969), 25.

DOCUMENT 13:

The Hippocratic *Oath*[13]

The *Oath* attributed to Hippocrates is certainly the best known of the Hippocratic writings, as it is still used in medical schools around the world. The text below represents possibly the earliest version of the *Oath*, which scholars have dated anywhere from the fifth century BCE to the second century CE. It provides a striking comparison to the previous Hippocratic sources, for it is primarily a religious document, an oath before the gods that the students of "Hippocrates" will set themselves apart, in terms of ethics and behavior, from their contemporary physicians.

ℰ

I swear by Apollo the physician, and Aesculapius, and Health [Hygieia], and All-heal [Panacea],[14] and all the gods and goddesses, that, according to my ability and judgment, I will keep this Oath and this stipulation—to reckon him who taught me this Art equally dear to me as my parents, to share my substance with him, and relieve his necessities if required; to look upon his offspring in the same footing as my own brothers, and to teach them this art, if they shall wish to learn it, without fee or stipulation; and that by precept, lecture, and every other mode of instruction, I will impart a knowledge of the Art to my own sons, and those of my teachers, and to disciples bound by a stipulation and oath according to the law of medicine, but to none others. I will follow that system of regimen which, according to my ability and judgment, I consider for the benefit of my patients, and abstain from whatever is deleterious and mischievous. I will give no deadly medicine to any one if asked, nor suggest any such counsel; and in like manner I will not give to a woman a **pessary** to produce abortion. With purity and with holiness I will pass my life and practice my Art. I will not cut persons **laboring under the stone**, but will leave this to be done by men who are practitioners of this work. Into whatever houses I enter, I will go into them for the benefit of the sick, and will abstain from every voluntary act of mischief and corruption; and, further from the seduction of females or males, of freemen and slaves. Whatever, in connection with my professional practice or not, in connection with it, I see or hear, in the life of men, which ought not to be spoken of abroad, I will not divulge, as reckoning that all such should be kept secret. While I continue to keep this Oath unviolated, may it be granted to me to enjoy life and the practice of the art, respected

pessary: A medicated tampon made of cotton, cloth, or some other absorbent substance for insertion in the vagina or rectum.

laboring under the stone: Suffering from kidney stones or bladder stones.

---

13 Francis Adams, *The Genuine Works of Hippocrates* (Dover, 1868).

14 Hygieia and Panacea were said to be two of the five daughters of Asclepius.

by all men, in all times! But should I trespass and violate this Oath, may the reverse be my lot!

DOCUMENT 14:
Pindar: Apollo Leaves Asclepius with Chiron the Centaur[15]

After Homer, Pindar (522–443 BCE) is one of the most famous poets from ancient Greece in the "Archaic Age" (eighth century BCE to ca. 480 BCE). His *epinikia*, or "victory odes," preserve many examples of Greek myths and religious belief, including the story of Asclepius and his medical knowledge.

ev

... Apollo spoke: "I can no longer endure in my soul to destroy my own child [Asclepius] by a most pitiful death, together with his mother's grievous suffering." So he spoke. In one step he reached the child and snatched it from the corpse; the burning fire divided its blaze for him, and he bore the child away and gave him to the **Magnesian Centaur** to teach him to heal many painful diseases for men. And those who came to him afflicted with congenital sores, or with their limbs wounded by gray bronze or by a far-hurled stone, or with their bodies wasting away from summer's fire or winter's cold, he released and delivered all of them from their different pains, tending some of them with gentle incantations, others with soothing potions, or by wrapping remedies all around their limbs, and others he set right with surgery.

Magnesian Centaur: Another name for Chiron the Centaur.

---

15   *The Odes of Pindar*, translated by Diane Arnson Svarlien, *Perseus Project* 1.0 (1991), 3.40–53. Available at perseus.tufts.edu.

DOCUMENT 15:

Celsus Celebrates Asclepius as a Man[16]

The Roman author Aulus Cornelius Celsus (ca. 25 BCE–ca. 50 CE) doubted whether Asclepius was actually a god. In his encyclopedia *De medicina* (*On Medicine*) he records the legendary history of why Asclepius, described here as a man and not a god, is celebrated as a medical authority.

e

Just as agriculture promises nourishment to healthy bodies, so does the Art of Medicine promise health to the sick. Nowhere is this Art wanting, for the most uncivilized nations have had knowledge of herbs, and other things to hand for the aiding of wounds and diseases. This Art, however, has been cultivated among the Greeks much more than in other nations—not, however, even among them from their first beginnings, but only for a few generations before ours. Hence Aesculapius is celebrated as the most ancient authority, and because he cultivated this science, as yet rude and vulgar, with a little more than common refinement, he was numbered among the gods. After him his two sons, Podalirius and Machaon, who followed Agamemnon as leader to the Trojan War, gave no inconsiderable help to their comrades. Homer stated, however, not that they gave any aid in the pestilence or in the various sorts of diseases, but only that they relieved wounds by the knife and by medicaments. Hence it appears that by them those parts only of the Art were attempted, and that they were the oldest. From the same authority, indeed, it can be learned that diseases were then ascribed to the anger of the immortal gods, and from them help used to be sought; and it is probable that with no aids against bad health, none the less health was generally good because of good habits, which neither indolence nor luxury had vitiated: since it is these two which have afflicted the bodies of men, first in Greece, and later amongst us; and hence this complex Art of Medicine, not needed in former times, nor among other nations even now, scarcely protracts the lives of a few of us to the verge of old age.

---

16   Celsus, *De Medicina*, translated by W.G. Spencer (Harvard UP, 1935–38).

DOCUMENT 16:

Greek Anatomical Votive Plaque of a Leg[17]

This sculpted plaque of a leg was left as a votive, or ritual offering, at a healing sanctuary in Melos in the years ca. 100–200 CE. The Greek inscription reads "Tyche [dedicated this] to Asclepius and Hygieia as a thank offering." Hygieia, the goddess of hygiene, was one of the five daughters of Asclepius in classical myth. Many votive plaques left for Asclepius represent the body part which was believed to have been helped by the god.

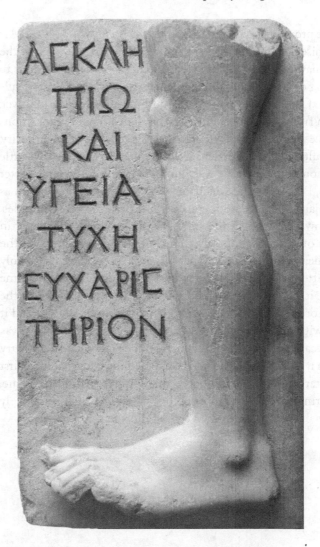

17 From the British Museum, photograph by Marie-Lan Nguyen.

DOCUMENT 17:

Aelius Aristides Dreams of Asclepius[18]

Aelius Aristides (117–181 CE) was a famous Roman orator and author, who traveled widely throughout the Roman Empire during its most prosperous period. He also was chronically ill, or thought he was, which we know from his detailed and highly stylized records of his illnesses, physicians, and treatments. He recorded this information in his *Sacred Tales*, written in short pieces over the years ca. 145–170 CE. He demonstrates how a learned Roman during the imperial era could seek both natural and religious remedies for illness.

℮

January 4 to February 15 166

But now I wish to indicate to you the condition of my abdomen. I shall reckon each matter day by day. It was the month of Poseidon, and what a winter it was! During those nights my stomach was upset and I had extraordinary insomnia, so that I could not digest the smallest morsel. Not the least cause was the continuous succession of stormy weather, which it was said even the tiling did not sustain. But I perspired all this time, except when I bathed.

January 4, 5, & 6

On the twelfth of the month, **the God** instructed me not to bathe, and the same on the next day, and the day after that. I passed these three days in a row, both night and day, wholly without perspiring, so that I did not even need to wear an undershirt, and never before did I perceive myself to be more comfortable. I passed the time in walking about the house and in games, as these were holidays. For the Vigil of the God followed upon the preceding holiday in honor of Poseidon.

the God: Asclepius.

January 7, Night & Day

And after this, there was a dream which contained a notion of bathing, although this was far from certain. *I dreamed that I had been in some way befouled.* Nevertheless I decided that I would bathe and that if I had actually

---

18   C.A. Behr, *Aelius Aristides and the Sacred Tales* (Amsterdam, 1968), 206–07, 211–12, 217–18. Italics within the text indicate diagnostic dreams.

experienced this befouling, there was need of water. And immediately thereafter I was somewhat uncomfortable in the bath and when I came out, everything seemed to be full and my breath was like that of a man gasping for air, so that right at the beginning I stopped taking nourishment. After this at night, stomach trouble, which reached such a pitch, that it scarcely stopped a little before noon. But there was a dream vision somewhat as follows: *I was in the warm bath, and bending forward I saw that my lower intestinal tract was in a rather strange state. I determined not to persist in not bathing. But someone said that the trouble which had appeared was not in the bathing itself and that I was not reasonable to guard against bathing as the cause.*

January 8

I bathed at evening and at dawn I had pains in my abdomen, and the pain spread over the right side down to the groin.

January 9, 10, & 11

On the **seventeenth no bathing after a dream, and on the eighteenth** no bathing. On the nineteenth, *I dreamed that some Parthians had got me in their power, and one of them approached me and made as if to brand me. Next he inserted a finger in my throat and poured in something, according to some native custom, and named it "indigestion." Later I recounted these things as they had appeared in the dream. And the audience marvelled and said that the cause of my thirst and inability to drink was this, that my food turned sour. Because of this **vomiting was indicated** and the Parthian ordered that I abstain from bathing today and produce one servant as a witness of this.* No bathing, and vomiting, and comfort....

February 13

On the next day, there was no bathing and vomiting of food. And when I vomited, my condition was such that I was glad if I could suffice for the day following.

February 14

On the day following, fasting was enjoined, but enjoined in this way. *I dreamed that I was in Smyrna, distrusting everything plain and visible, because I was not aware that I had made the journey. Figs were offered to me. Next the prophet Corus was present and showed that there was a quick acting poison in them. After this, I was full of suspicion and eagerly vomited, and at the same time considered what if I should not have vomited completely? Next someone said that there was also some poison in some other figs. Therefore I was still more distressed and angry because I did not hear it sooner.* After these things were seen, I suspected that fasting was indicated, but if not, still I preferred it. But I asked the God to show more clearly what he meant, fasting or vomiting.

I slept again and *I thought I was in the Temple of Pergamum and that now the middle of the day had passed and I was fasting. And* **Theodotus** *came to me with some friends, and having entered, he sat down beside me while I was lying thus upon the couch. I said to him that I was fasting. But he indicated that he knew, and said that "after all the things which these men are doing, I have put off performing a* **phlebotomy** *on you. For there is an aggravation of the kidneys and fasting," he said, "is sort of a bastard outlet, which goes through the chest, for the inflammation." And while he said this, two sparks appeared before me. And in wonder I looked at Theodotus and felt it an omen of his words, and I asked him what these were. He said that they were from the inflammation, and he indicated what was troubling me.* Then I awoke, and I found that it was that very hour, in which I thought that Theodotus spoke to me, and friends had actually now come to visit me.

These dreams appeared to me while the doctor had arrived and had prepared himself to help, as much as he knew how. But when he heard the dreams, being a sensible man, he also yielded to the God. And we recognized the true and proper doctor for us, and we did what he commanded.

February 15

Now my night was comfortable in every way and everything was without pain.

Theodotus: Aristides' former doctor, long dead by the time of this account in 166 CE.

phlebotomy: Cutting into a vein for the purpose of medical bloodletting, usually to balance the humors. Also called venesection.

DOCUMENT 18:
An Egyptian God in Greco-Roman Dress: Imouthes as Asclepius[19]

> This document was written in Roman Egypt sometime in the first to the
> sixth centuries CE. It records the anonymous Egyptian author's vision of
> Imouthes, or Imhotep, the Egyptian god of physicians. Imhotep may have
> been a real person, the chancellor to the pharaoh around 2700 BCE, but he
> was later deified for his great wisdom. It was only many centuries later that
> Imhotep was venerated as a god of healing, possibly under the influence of
> the cult of Asclepius. This influence is clearly seen below, in which the author
> describes Imouthes coming in a dream much like Asclepius.

It was night, when every living creature was asleep except those in pain,
but divinity showed itself the more effectively; a violent fever burned me,
and I was convulsed with loss of breath and coughing, owing to the pain
proceeding from my side. Heavy in the head with my troubles I was lapsing
half-conscious into sleep, and my mother, as a mother would for her child
(and she is by nature affectionate), being extremely grieved at my agonies
was sitting without enjoying even a short period of slumber, when suddenly
she perceived—it was no dream or sleep, for her eyes were open immovably,
though not seeing clearly, for a divine and terrifying vision came to her, easily
preventing her from observing the god himself or his servants, whichever
it was. In any case there was someone whose height was more than human,
clothed in shining raiment and carrying in his left hand a book, who after
merely regarding me two or three times from head to foot disappeared.
When she had recovered herself, she tried, still trembling, to wake me, and
finding that the fever had left me and that much sweat was pouring off me,
did reverence to the manifestation of the god, and then wiped me and made
me more collected. When I spoke with her, she wished to declare the virtue
of the god, but I anticipating her told her all myself; for everything that she
saw in the vision appeared to me in dreams. After these pains in my side had
ceased and the god had given me yet another assuaging cure, I proclaimed
his benefits. But when we had again besought his favors by sacrifices to
the best of our ability, he demanded through the priest who serves him in
the ceremonies the fulfillment of the promise long ago announced to him,
and we, although knowing ourselves to be debtors in neither sacrifices nor
votive offering, nevertheless supplicated him again with them. But when he

---

19 Bernard P. Grenfell and Arthur S. Hunt, translators, *The Oxyrhyncus Papyri*, Part XI (London, 1915),
    no. 1381, 230–31.

said repeatedly that he cared not for these but for what had been previously promised, I was at a loss, and with difficulty, since I disparaged it, felt the divine obligation of the composition. But since thou hadst once noticed, master, that I was neglecting the divine book, invoking thy providence and filled with thy divinity I hastened to the inspired task of the history. And I hope to extend by my proclamation the fame of thy inventiveness; for I unfolded truly by a physical treatise in another book the convincing account of the creation of the world. Throughout the composition I have filled up defects and struck out superfluities, and in telling a rather long tale I have spoken briefly and narrated once for all a complicated story. Hence, master, I conjecture that the book has been completed in accordance with thy favour, not with my aim; for such a record in writing suits thy divinity. And as the discoverer of this art, Asclepius, greatest of gods and my teacher, thou are distinguished by the thanks of all men. For every gift of a votive offering or sacrifice lasts only for the immediate moment, and presently perishes, while a written record is an undying gift of gratitude, from time to time renewing its youth in the memory. Every Greek tongue will tell thy story, and every Greek man will worship the son of **Ptah**, Imouthes. Assemble hither, ye kindly and good men; avaunt ye malignant and impious! Assemble all ye, who by serving the god have been cured of diseases, ye who practice the healing art, ye who will labor as zealous followers of virtue, ye who have been blessed by great abundance of benefits, ye who have been saved from the dangers of the sea! For every place has been perpetrated by the saving power of the god.

Ptah: One of the most ancient Egyptian creator gods, patron of craftsmen and architects, as well as the supposed father of Imhotep.

PART 3

Professional Medicine in the Roman Mediterranean (ca. 1–300 CE)

The physician and philosopher Galen of Pergamon (ca. 130–ca. 210 CE) was the most famous advocate for the incorporation of Hippocratic medicine into Roman culture, even though Hippocratic ideas had been influencing Roman culture since the later Roman Republican period (ca. 200–27 BCE). Galen was Greek by language and culture, but he was very much a child of the Roman Empire, born in a vibrant Roman colonial city (Pergamon, now outside modern Bergama, Turkey) and eventually serving in Rome as a gladiator physician and then imperial physician to Marcus Aurelius (r. 161–180 CE), a deeply learned emperor. Galen was one of the most productive authors in the Greek language, writing hundreds of treatises on medicine, anatomy, psychology, philosophy, ethics, and even linguistics. His extant writings form at least ten percent of all surviving classical Greek literature. He wrote two catalogues of his works (*My Own Books* and *The Order of My Own Books*) as a guideline to readers of where to begin and as a protection against the works falsely attributed to him even during his own lifetime. Galen wrote works on anatomy, therapeutics, and prognosis; numerous commentaries on Hippocratic works; criticisms of earlier physicians like Erasistratus (304–250 BCE) and Asclepiades of Bithynia (129–40 BCE) and of the Empiric and Methodist sects (schools of medical theory); philosophical works on logical proofs, morals, the works of Plato and Aristotle, as well as on Epicurus and the Stoics. He wrote some of his medical works in a simpler form for students, such as *Sects for Beginners*, *Bones for Beginners*, and *Pulse for Beginners*. The scope of his works shows that he tried to balance being a philosopher and a doctor, two careers that were often seen in his day as irreconcilable, because a good philosopher was not supposed to work with his hands as doctors did. Galen wrote a short work on finding this balance: *The Best Doctor Is also a Philosopher*.

In many of his works, Galen sought to establish Hippocratic humoralism as the only valid medical system and to promote himself as the best interpreter of that system. This is evident in *On the Medical Sects* (Document 19) in which Galen analyzes (with obvious bias) the various schools of medicine supposedly active in his time: the Dogmatists, Empiricists, Methodists, Pneumatists, and Eclectics. Galen's favorable description of the Dogmatists and Empiricists matches most closely with the ideas in the major Hippocratic texts and in his own works. Clearly not every physician agreed with Hippocratic humoralism, or with the idea that one overarching theory could apply to all patients, but the adherents of all five of the aforementioned sects agreed that the causes of disease and healing were natural and thus could be rationalized and taught. Galen also shows his devotion to Hippocrates in his treatise *On Black Bile* (Document 25) along with a willingness to go beyond specific aspects of Hippocratic medicine to craft his own more rigorous system of humoral theory.

Classical medical authors discussed not only general theories of disease causation but also the nature and treatment of specific diseases. We must remember, however, that while many of their terms for diseases are the same as ours today (pneumonia, tetanus, epilepsy, migraine), our understanding of their causes is significantly different. In Document 20, we see an example of how a predecessor of Galen, Aretaeus the Cappadocian (first century CE), author of *Causes and Symptoms of Acute Diseases*, understood the disease of tetanus. Aretaeus provides both a clinical description of tetanus and a poignant account of the patient's agonies and the physician's difficulties in treating this condition. He claims that tetanus is incurable (which it was before modern antibiotics and antitoxins), but this admission is rare among ancient physicians. Although Aretaeus gives due credit to Hippocrates in his writings, he rarely adopts the humoral theory and practiced a more hands-on and invasive form of medicine than Hippocratic-Galenic physicians. A contemporary of Aretaeus, Rufus of Ephesus provided instructions and examples of a physician's bedside manner during diagnosis and prognosis. Rufus was active around 100 CE and wrote numerous medical works, including his *Medical Questions* (Document 21). He describes in a frank manner how a physician must address and question a patient. Rufus was a great admirer of Hippocrates, but not afraid to differ from the great authority, as he indicates.

Roughly contemporary with Rufus was the author Celsus, who wrote his eight-book work *De medicina* (*On Medicine*, Document 22) as a summary of learned medicine for Latin readers. He probably was not a practicing physician, but clearly had a firm grasp of medical practice and theory. *De medicina* is the only surviving section of a monumental encyclopedia on the major trades and arts in the early Roman Empire, including agriculture, war, rhetoric, law, and philosophy. In *De medicina*, Celsus lays out practical instructions for maintaining health and preventing disease without the aid of physicians. These include a common-sense and self-managed regimen of diet, exercise, sexual intercourse, and a life of moderation.

The primary treatments for disease in the ancient and medieval world took the form of plant-based remedies. Such cures are mentioned throughout ancient medical literature, from the Ebers Papyrus (Document 2, pp. 15–16) to the Hippocratic Corpus and the writings of Galen. The collected information about the medicinal action of plants (what we now call "pharmacy") was gathered into "herbals" by several classical authors, most famously by the Greco-Roman physician and soldier Pedanios Dioscorides (ca. 40–90 CE). His work *De materia medica* (its Latin title) served as the basis for most Western pharmacology for the next 15 centuries. Dioscorides' herbal (Document 23) was widely known throughout Europe and the Mediterranean in the Middle Ages, when it was translated into Latin and Arabic, and expanded and edited to include new herbal substances. John Riddle, the modern expert on Dioscorides, outlines the 12 thematic elements found in most of the approximately 600 entries in *De materia medica*:

1) Name of plant and synonyms; 2) Habitat; 3) Botanical description; 4) Drug properties or actions; 5) Medicinal usages; 6) Harmful side effects; 7) Quantities and dosages; 8) Harvesting, preparation, and storage instructions; 9) Adulteration methods and tests for detection; 10) Veterinary usages; 11) Magical and nonmedical usages; 12) Specific geographical locations or habitats.[1]

No single passage contains all 12 of these elements, but many of them are found in most entries. His book was not just a list of plants, but a detailed and practical medical manual.

Galen not only elaborated the medical theory of Hippocrates, but also reported in detail his experience as a practicing physician to promote his own reputation. In several works, he relates stories of his skill as a physician, teacher, and philosopher, such as in his treatise *On the Affected Places* (Document 24). He boasts of a seemingly magical ability to make "diagnoses and prognoses which approach to divination rather than to the art of medicine." In a similar famous passage from *On Prognosis*, Galen records how he cured Emperor Marcus Aurelius of a feverish paroxysm after many other physicians failed. In these stories Galen dramatizes his ability to diagnose difficult diseases, as he acts like an ancient Sherlock Holmes, organizing obscure clues into a satisfying medical narrative.

The dietary regimens and herbal treatments of Hippocrates, Galen, and other Greco-Roman physicians were intended mostly for run-of-the-mill illnesses, affecting individual patients. Epidemic diseases, which destroyed entire populations, were far more difficult to treat using the dominant

---

1 John M. Riddle, *Dioscorides on Pharmacy and Medicine* (U of Texas P, 2011), 25–27.

humoral medical theory, and classical authors turned more readily to the gods to understand them and looked for novel explanations of their source. For example; Livy (Titus Livius, 59 BCE–17 CE) described in his *History of Rome* how a plague (possibly malaria, typhus, anthrax, or a comorbidity of these diseases[2]) struck the Romans in the fifth century BCE while they were fighting their neighbors, the Volscians and Aequi. The Roman senate and the matrons of Rome all implored the gods to end the pestilence. Livy, however, compares these religious reactions to the natural medical theories of his own day when he concludes, "Whether it was that the gods graciously answered prayer or that the unhealthy season had passed, people gradually threw off the influence of the epidemic and the public health became more satisfactory."[3] Natural explanations for epidemic diseases are also evident in the historian Herodian of Antioch's description of the "Antonine Plague," which struck the Roman Empire in the years ca. 165–180 CE (Document 26). This "plague" was most likely smallpox or measles, but the pathogen has yet to be identified for certain. Herodian describes how Commodus, co-emperor with his father Marcus Aurelius for the years 177–180 CE, avoided getting sick. The Roman doctors prescribed sweet smells and perfumes to block the polluted air which was believed to spread the plague (essentially the same explanation given by physicians for the later medieval Black Death).

2   Scarborough, *Roman Medicine*, 16.

3   Livy, *The History of Rome*, translated by Rev. Canon Roberts, Vol. 1, Everyman's Library (J.M. Dent & Sons, 1905), 3.7–8.

Galen, *On the Medical Sects*[4]

> *On the Medical Sects* was one of Galen of Pergamon's (ca. 130–210 CE) most
> influential works in shaping both the medieval and modern understanding
> of ancient medicine. In it he describes and dismisses most of the "schools"
> or "sects" of medical thought that had developed and spread throughout the
> eastern Mediterranean during the Hellenistic and Roman eras up to his date.
> These groups probably did not exist as coherent "schools" but rather reflect
> Galen's own views on the different types of medical theory.

℘

II [*Empiricists*]. Now, the Empiricists for their part say that the medical art
arose in the following manner. Many **affections** were observed occurring in
people, some spontaneously, both in healthy and unhealthy subjects—for
instance, a bleeding at the nose, an access of sweating, diarrhœa or any other
similar affection, which prove either harmful or advantageous, but which
was produced by no obvious cause. Of others, again, the cause might be
evident, albeit independent of any choice on our own part, and taking place
as it were by chance; for example, it might happen that when a person fell
down, or was struck or wounded in any way, he would bleed; or again, if sick,
he might, in obedience to his instincts, drink cold water, or wine or the like,
each of which things might prove either advantageous or the reverse. The first
of these beneficial or harmful happenings the Empiricists call natural, and
the second, fortuitous. To one's first meeting with either of these the term
accidental encounter is applied, from the fact of their occurring by chance,
and independently of volition.

> **affections:** Any medical condition.

Such, then, is the *accidental* type of experience. What is called *improvised
experience* is when one deliberately tests something that has been suggested
by dreams or the like.

Further, there is also a third kind of experience, the *imitative*, in which
something which, occurring either by nature, chance, or improvisation, has
proved helpful or the reverse, is tested anew in the same diseases by *experi-
ment*; this it is upon which the art of the Empiricists is mainly based; for,
after having imitated, *not once, nor twice, but repeatedly*, the treatment which
proved salutary on a former occasion, and having found that, for the most
part, it has the same action in the same affections, they give to the record of

---

4   Arthur J. Brock, *Greek Medicine, Being Extracts Illustrative of Medical Writers from Hippocrates to
    Galen* (J.M. Dent & Sons, 1929), 130–51: 132–36, 140–41.

a fact like this the name *theorem*, deeming it now to be worthy of reliance, and to form an integral portion of the medical art.

And when they have gathered together a number of such theorems the whole collection is known as Medicine, and the collector as a Physician. Such a collection is also called by them an **autopsy**, being, as it were, a record of things frequently observed to happen in the same manner. They also term it an *experience*, and the record of it a **history**; the same thing, in fact, is an autopsy from the observer's point of view, and a history from that of the student to whom it is related....

III [*Rationalists or Dogmatists*]. Now, the method which proceeds by way of *reflection* or *reasoning* advises a thorough study of the *nature* of the body which we are endeavouring to heal, as well as the properties of all those factors from daily exposure to which the body becomes of itself more healthy or more sickly. Next after this, they say the physician must be acquainted with **airs, waters, localities**, occupations, food, drink, and customs, so that he may discover on the one hand the causes of all diseases, and with respect to remedies on the other hand may be able both to compare their properties and to reckon how any given one of them, having such and such a property, will, when applied to such and such a pathogenic factor, have naturally such and such an effect.

Until he has a broad training in all these matters, say the Dogmatists, he cannot possibly have success with his remedies. For instance—in order that you may see the whole by means of a small example—suppose a part of the body to be painful, hard, resistant, and increased in bulk; here the physician must first investigate the cause which has determined the inflow of fluid in abnormal quantity into the part, the latter being thereby swollen, stretched, and rendered painful. Next, if the fluid be still gathering, he must check it, or, if not, he must proceed to empty the part.

How, then, are you to stop the continued influx, and evacuate what has already collected? You will check the inflow by **refrigerants** and **styptics**, and you will empty the matter which has already collected by warming and relaxing the part.

Thus the Rationalists obtain from the condition itself the *indication* of the appropriate remedy; yet they say that this is not enough by itself, but that another indication is obtained from the strength of the patient, another from his age, and another from his personal nature; also that special indications for treatment are afforded by the season of the year, the nature of the locality, and from occupations and customs.

Thus—in order that you may learn this further point more clearly from an example—let us suppose an individual to be acutely fevered, shrinking from all movement, and oppressed by the weight of his body; suppose him

autopsy: From the Greek for "personal observation," a broader term than our modern "autopsy."

history: Our word "history" does indeed come originally from a term (Greek *istoria*, Latin *historia*) used for written records of medical or scientific observations.

airs, waters, localities: A reference to the Hippocratic work *Airs, Waters, Places* (Document 11, pp. 42–45).

refrigerants: Medications and medical procedures used by the Dogmatists to cool the body and slow the influx of excess fluid.

styptics: Like modern styptics, which are medicating agents designed to restrict blood flow and seal injured blood vessels, the styptic medicines of the Dogmatists were prescribed to constrict the flow of any fluid in the body.

also to be more congested and more red than usual, and even his veins to stand out more prominently. It is surely plain to everybody that such an one has a plethora of over-heated blood. What, then, is the cure? Clearly evacuation, since this is the opposite of plethora, and *opposites are the cure for opposites*. How, then, are we to evacuate this, and to what extent? This question cannot be determined by the cause alone; we must also have regard to the patient's strength and age, the season, the locality, and all the other considerations just mentioned. Thus if he be strong and in the prime of life, and if the season be spring and the region temperate, you cannot go wrong in opening a vein and letting out as much blood as the condition demands; but if the patient be weak, or quite a small child, or a very old man, and if the region be a cold one, as in the neighborhood of Scythia, or torrid, as in that of Ethiopia, and if the season of the year be either very hot or very cold—under these circumstances nobody would venture to carry out **venesection**. In the same way also Rationalists bid us consider customs, occupations, and the physiological condition in each case, since from all of these is to be obtained a special indication for the appropriate treatment.

venesection: Cutting into a vein for the purpose of medical bloodletting to balance the humors. Also called phlebotomy.

[In chapters IV and V, Galen proceeds to compare the methods of Dogmatists and Empiricists and the disputes between these two "schools" of medicine, before proceeding to heap scorn on his avowed enemies the Methodists.]

VI [*Methodists*]. Now, those called Methodists—for they give themselves this name on the ground that even their predecessors, the Dogmatists, denied using method in Medicine—the Methodists, I say, seem to me not only to dispute the ancient teachings in the matter of rationale, but to make many alterations in the actual practice of the art. They say, in fact, that nothing useful as regards *indications for treatment* is to be got either from the part affected, the immediate cause, the time of life, the season or locality, nor from an investigation of the patient's strength, nature, or bodily habit. Further, they will hear nothing of *customs*, but they affirm that they derive sufficient indication for treatment from *the diseases themselves*—and these not considered each as a separate entity, but on more broad and general lines. Moreover they give the name of "communities" to those same general principles, which pervade all particular conditions; and they try to demonstrate that there are merely two such communities and a third or mixed kind—some say only in those diseases which come within the province of regimen, and others say in all diseases. To these communities they give the name of *obstruction* and *flux*; every malady, they say, is either obstructed or fluent, or else a combination of the two. If the natural evacuations of the body are checked, they call this an obstructed condition, and if they are escaping somewhat too freely, they call this fluent; when they are both checked and fluent, they say that a *complex* exists; thus, for instance, in an eye which is at once inflamed and discharging, they say that, since inflammation, which is "a disease of obstruction," occurs here not by itself but simultaneously with and in the same place as discharge, this makes the whole process a "complected" disease.

Now the remedy indicated in diseases of obstruction is relaxation.... For example, they say that, if the knee be inflamed, we must relax it; if the bowels or eye be running, we must check and repress them. In complected states we must stop the more urgent of the two elements; it is, in fact, the one which is giving the most trouble and which involves danger—that is, the stronger one—that must be opposed rather than the other ...

[In chapters VII–IX Galen attempts to demolish the reputation of the Methodists using logic and invective. He poses as both an Empiricist and a Dogmatist to criticize the Methodists' over-simplification of medical diagnosis and treatment.]

DOCUMENT 20:

Aretaeus the Cappadocian on the Difficult Case of Tetanus[5]

> Aretaeus was a Greek physician in the Roman Empire during the first century CE. He wrote numerous works on the diagnosis and treatment of different diseases, and is recognized as going far beyond the Hippocratics in providing detailed clinical descriptions of epilepsy, asthma, cancer, and other conditions. In the passage below, Aretaeus describes the causes and symptoms of tetanus, differentiates its varieties, and provides a heart-breaking account of the torturous pain it causes.

Tetanus, in all its varieties, is a spasm of an exceedingly painful nature, very swift to prove fatal, but neither easy to be removed. They are affections of the muscles and tendons about the jaws; but the illness is communicated to the whole frame, for all parts are affected sympathetically with the primary organs. There are three forms of the convulsion, namely, in a straight line, backwards, and forwards. Tetanus is in a direct line, when the person laboring under the distention is stretched out straight and inflexible. The contractions forwards and backwards have their appellation from the tension and the place; for that backwards we call *Opisthotonos*; and that variety we call *Emprosthotonos* in which the patient is bent forwards by the anterior nerves. For the Greek word *TONOS* is applied both to a nerve, and to signify tension.

Opisthotonos ... Emprosthotonos: Greek terms for "tension behind" and "tension brought forward," which are still used in modern medicine to refer to types of tetanic spasm.

The causes of these complaints are many; for some are apt to supervene on the wound of a membrane, or of muscles, or of punctured nerves, when, for the most part, the patients die; for "spasm from a wound is fatal." And women also suffer from this spasm after abortion; and, in this case, they seldom recover. Others are attacked with the spasm owing to a severe blow in the neck. Severe cold also sometimes proves a cause; for this reason, winter of all the seasons most especially engenders these affections; next to it, spring and autumn, but least of all summer, unless when preceded by a wound, or when any strange diseases prevail epidemically. Women are more disposed to tetanus than men, because they are of a cold temperament; but they more readily recover, because they are of a humid. With respect to the different ages, children are frequently affected, but do not often die, because the affection is familiar and akin to them; striplings are less liable to suffer, but more readily die; adults least of all, whereas old men are most

---

5 Aretaeus, *Causes and Symptoms of Acute Diseases* I.6, from *The Extant Works of Aretaeus, the Cappadocian*, translated by Francis Adams (1856).

subject to the disease, and most apt to die; the cause of this is the frigidity and dryness of old age, and the nature of the death. But if the cold be along with humidity, these spasmodic diseases are more innocent, and attended with less danger.

In all these varieties, then, to speak generally, there is a pain and tension of the tendons and spine, and of the muscles connected with the jaws and cheek; for they fasten the lower jaw to the upper, so that it could not easily be separated even with levers or a wedge. But if one, by forcibly separating the teeth, pour in some liquid, the patients do not drink it but squirt it out, or retain it in the mouth, or it regurgitates by the nostrils; for the *isthmus faucium* is strongly compressed, and the tonsils being hard and tense, do not coalesce so as to propel that which is swallowed. The face is ruddy, and of mixed colors, the eyes almost immoveable, or are rolled about with difficulty; strong feeling of suffocation; respiration bad, distension of the arms and legs; *subsultus* of the muscles; the countenance variously distorted; the cheeks and lips tremulous; the jaw quivering, and the teeth rattling, and in certain rare cases even the ears are thus affected. I myself have beheld this and wondered! The urine is retained, so as to induce strong **dysuria**, or passes spontaneously from contraction of the bladder. These symptoms occur in each variety of the spasms.

But there are peculiarities in each; in Tetanus there is tension in a straight line of the whole body, which is unbent and inflexible; the legs and arms are straight.

Opisthotonos bends the patient backward, like a bow, so that the reflected head is lodged between the shoulder-blades; the throat protrudes; the jaw sometimes gapes, but in some rare cases it is fixed in the upper one; respiration stertorous; the belly and chest prominent, and in these there is usually incontinence of urine; the abdomen stretched, and resonant if tapped; the arms strongly bent back in a state of extension; the legs and thighs are bent together, for the legs are bent in the opposite direction to the hams.

But if they are bent forwards, they are protuberant at the back, the loins being extruded in a line with the back, the whole of the spine being straight; the vertex prone, the head inclining towards the chest; the lower jaw fixed upon the breast bone; the hands clasped together, the lower extremities extended; pains intense; the voice altogether dolorous; they groan, making deep moaning. Should the mischief then seize the chest and the respiratory organs, it readily frees the patient from life; a blessing this, to himself, as being a deliverance from pains, distortion, and deformity; and a contingency less than usual to be lamented by the spectators, were he a son or a father. But should the powers of life still stand out, the respiration, although bad, being still prolonged, the patient is not only bent up into an arch but rolled together like a ball, so that the head rests upon the knees, while the legs and

isthmus faucium: The upper part of the throat, near the tonsils (still the term used today).

subsultus: Involuntary twitching.

dysuria: Painful and difficult urination.

back are bent forwards, so as to convey the impression of the articulation of the knee being dislocated backwards.

An inhuman calamity! an unseemly sight! a spectacle painful even to the beholder! an incurable malady! owing to the distortion, not to be recognized by the dearest friends; and hence the prayer of the spectators, which formerly would have been reckoned not pious, now becomes good, that the patient may depart from life, as being a deliverance from the pains and unseemly evils attendant on it. But neither can the physician, though present and looking on, furnish any assistance, as regards life, relief from pain or from deformity. For if he should wish to straighten the limbs, he can only do so by cutting and breaking those of a living man. With them, then, who are overpowered by the disease, he can merely sympathize. This is the great misfortune of the physician.

DOCUMENT 21:

Rufus of Ephesus, *Medical Questions*: Interrogation of the Patient[6]

> Rufus of Ephesus was a Greek physician in the Roman empire, active around
> 100 CE. He wrote numerous medical works, including *Medical Questions*.
> He describes in a frank manner how a physician must address and question
> a patient. Rufus was a great admirer of Hippocrates, but not afraid to differ
> from his authority.

~

One must put questions to the patient, for thereby certain aspects of the disease can be better understood, and the treatment rendered more effective. And I place the interrogation of the patient himself first, since in this way you can learn how far his mind is healthy or otherwise; also his physical strength and weakness; and you can get some idea of the disease and the part affected. For, if his answers are given in a consecutive way, and from memory, and are relevant, and if he shows no hesitancy either in judgment or utterance; if he answers according to his natural bent; that is to say, if, being in other ways well-bred, he answers gently and politely; or if, on the other hand, being naturally bold or timid, he answers in a bold or timid way, one may then look on him as being at least sound mentally. But if you ask him one thing and he answers another; and if in the middle of speaking his memory fails him; if, again, his enunciation is tremulous and hesitating and he exhibits complete changes of manner; all these are signs of mental inadequacy. In this way one also appreciates deafness in a patient; if he does not hear, one must in addition inquire of those about him whether he was in any way deaf before, or whether it is the disease that has made him so. This is a very important diagnostic point....

And suppose someone says that my methods of inquiry are contrary to those of **Hippocrates**, who claims to have discovered the art by which a physician, on arriving at a city unfamiliar to him, may find out about the water, the seasons, the condition of the inhabitants' digestive organs, whether they are much given to eating and drinking, what diseases are ordinarily endemic, and how the women manage in childbirth; and there are various other matters which this authority undertakes to find out personally by means of his Art, without putting any questions to the natives. If, I say, anyone brings this forward and reproaches me for not agreeing with the greatest of physicians on such all-important matters, my answer is that I do not despise any of the work of Hippocrates; I certainly hold that by

Hippocrates: Rufus is referring here to the Hippocratic work *Airs, Waters, Places* (Document 11, pp. 42–45).

6   A.J. Brock, translator, *Greek Medicine* (London, 1929), 113, 123–24.

his method also certain discoveries have been made about the state of the seasons, the constitution of the body, about various regimens, about the ordinary qualities and defects of waters and the general principles of disease. But I maintain that for diagnosis one also needs to procure information from the people of the place, especially in regard to anything strange and unusual in their countries. I admire Hippocrates for his ingenious method; undoubtedly a great many fine discoveries have been made by it. At the same time, I advise anyone wishing for an exact knowledge in these various matters not to neglect the method of interrogation.

DOCUMENT 22:

Celsus: A Healthy Regimen without Doctors[7]

Celsus (ca. 25 BCE–ca. 50 CE) wrote *De medicina* (*On Medicine*) as a summary of learned (i.e., Greek) medicine for Latin readers. He lays out practical instructions (a *regimen*) for maintaining health and preventing disease without the aid of physicians, including therapeutic bathing and a moderate diet and lifestyle.

❦

I.1. A man in health, who is both vigorous and his own master, should be under no obligatory rules, and have no need, either for a medical attendant, or for a **rubber and anointer**. His kind of life should afford him variety; he should be now in the country, now in town, and more often about the farm; he should sail, hunt, rest sometimes, but more often take exercise; for whilst inaction weakens the body, work strengthens it; the former brings on premature old age, the latter prolongs youth.

It is well also at times to go to the bath, at times to make use of cold waters; to undergo sometimes **inunction**, sometimes to neglect that same; to avoid no kind of food in common use; to attend at times a banquet, at times to hold aloof; to eat more than sufficient at one time, at another no more; to take food twice rather than once a day, and always as much as one wants provided one digests it. But whilst exercise and food of this sort are necessities, those of the athletes are redundant; for in the one class any break in the routine of exercise, owing to necessities of civil life, affects the body injuriously, and in the other, bodies thus fed up in their fashion age very quickly and become infirm.

Sexual intercourse indeed is neither to be desired overmuch, nor overmuch to be feared; seldom used it braces the body, used frequently it relaxes. Since, however, nature and not number should be the standard of frequency, regard being had to age and constitution, sexual intercourse can be recognized as harmless when followed neither by languor nor by pain. The use is worse in the day-time, and safer by night; but care should be taken that by day it be not immediately followed by a meal, and at night not immediately followed by work and watching. Such are the precautions to be observed by the strong, and they should take care that whilst in health their defences against ill-health are not used up.

I.2. The weak, however, among whom are a large portion of townspeople, and almost all those fond of letters, need greater precaution, so that care may

rubber and anointer: These are two of the attendants available in the larger Roman bathhouses. Celsus considers their skills unnecessary to the healthy man.

inunction: Anointing or rubbing with oil as part of the bathing experience.

---

7   Celsus, *De Medicina*, translated by W.G. Spencer (Harvard UP, 1935–38), I.1–2, II.17.

re-establish what the character of their constitution or of their residence or of their study detracts. Anyone therefore of these who has digested well may with safety rise early; if too little, he must stay in bed, or if he has been obliged to get up early, must go to sleep again; he who has not digested, should lie up altogether, and neither work nor take exercise nor attend to business. He who without heartburn eructates undigested food should drink cold water at intervals and none the less exercise self-control.

He should also reside in a house that is light, airy in summer, sunny in winter; avoid the midday sun, the morning and evening chill, also exhalations from rivers and marshes; and he should not often expose himself when the sky is cloudy to a sun that breaks through..., lest he should be affected alternately by cold and heat—a thing which excites particularly choked nostrils and running colds. Much more indeed are these things to be watched in unhealthy localities, where they even produce pestilence.

He can tell that his body is sound, if his morning urine is whitish, later reddish; the former indicates that digestion is going on, the latter that digestion is complete. On waking one should lie still for a while, then, except in winter time, bathe the face freely with cold water; when the days are long the siesta should be taken before the midday meal, when short, after it. In winter, it is best to rest in bed the whole night long; if there must be study by lamp-light, it should not be immediately after taking food, but after digestion. He who has been engaged in the day, whether in domestic or on public affairs, ought to keep some portion of the day for the care of the body. The primary care in this respect is exercise, which should always precede the taking of food; the exercise should be ampler in the case of one who has laboured less and digested less well.

II.17. Sweating also is elicited in two ways, either by dry heat, or by the bath. The dry is the heat of hot sand, of the **Laconian sweating-room**, and of the dry oven, and of some natural sweating places, where hot vapour exhaling from the ground is confined within a building, as we have it in the myrtle groves above Baiae. Besides these it is also derived from the sun and through exercise. These treatments are useful whenever humor is doing harm inside, and has to be dispersed. And also some diseases of sinews are best treated thus. But the other treatments may suit the infirm: sun and exercise only the more robust, who must, however, be free from fever, whether only at the commencement of a disease, or when actually in the grasp of a grave malady. But care must be taken that none of the above are tried either during fever or with food undigested.

Laconian sweating-room: A dry sweating-room in large Roman bathhouses, the invention of which was attributed to the Spartans (Laconians), who were believed by Romans not to have taken any other kind of bath.

DOCUMENT 23:
Dioscorides and the Science of Pharmacology[8]

> The Greco-Roman physician and soldier Pedanios Dioscorides (ca. 40–90 CE) compiled his herbal *De materia medica* based on his extensive travels with the military around the Mediterranean. It served as the basis for most European and Islamicate pharmacology for the next 15 centuries. He treats about 600 different plants, organized into five books. These include exotic spices, common herbs, and garden vegetables, as seen in the excerpts below.

ℰ

I.13. Cassia

There are many kinds of cassia that are grown in spice-bearing Arabia. It has thick-barked twigs, leaves similar to those of pepper. Select that which is pale yellow, fresh, and healthy looking, resembling coral, slender, long, and hard, like shepherd's pipe, bitter in taste, astringent with much fiery quality, aromatic, and like wine in smell. Such it is called by the inhabitants of the country by the name of *achy*, but is named *daphnitis* by the merchants in Alexandria. Better than this one is the dark, purple, thick kind called *gizir*, having a smell like a rose, most suitable for medicinal usages and the kind mentioned not often coming before the first-mentioned kind. The third kind is called *Mosulitis Gatos*. The other kinds are of inferior quality, such as that which is called *asuphe*, black with thin bark, and burst bark, also those kinds called *kitto* and *darka*.

There is also a kind of false cassia, unspeakable in resemblance, which is proven false by taste neither sharp nor aromatic, and it has a bark holding fast to it to the innermost part. One discovers broad tubes, soft, light, well sprouting, making a difference from the other kind. But reject that which is whitened beforehand and scabby and having a goatlike smell, and does not have a thick tube but strong and thin.

It has a diuretic, warming, drying, gently astringent quality. It is suitable as medicine for making the eyes sharp and as an emollient; with honey it removes moles; it brings out the menses and drunk it helps those with spider bites and also being drunk it is good for internal inflammations and inflammations of the kidneys and for women either as a sitz bath or as a fumigant it dilates the uterus. If cinnamon should be lacking then double

---

8   John M. Riddle, *Dioscorides on Pharmacy and Medicine* (U of Texas P, 1985), 25–27, 100. Translations adapted.

the amount of the medicine, it will do the same as cinnamon. It is very useful for many things.

II.136. Lettuce

Cultivated lettuce; good for upper tract, a little cooling, sleep causing, softening to lower tract, increasing lactation. Boiled down it increases nutrition. Unwashed and eaten it is given for upper digestive troubles. Its seeds being drunk are good for those who continually dream and they avert sexual intercourse; eaten too often they cause dim-sightedness. They are preserved in brine. The stalk growing up has something like the potency of the juice and sap of wild lettuce.

Wild lettuce; is similar to the cultivated, larger stalk; leaves: whiter, thinner, more rough, and bitter to taste. To some degree its properties are similar to those of opium poppy, thus some people mix its juice with opium. Whence its sap 2 **obols** in weight with sour wine purges away watery humors through the digestive tract; it cleans away **albugo**, misty eyes. It assists against the burning of eyes anointed on with woman's milk. Generally it is sleep inducing and anodyne. It expels the menses; it is given in a drink for scorpion and venomous spider bites. The seeds, similar to that of the cultivated kind, when drunk avert dreams and sexual intercourse. Its juice produces the same things but with a weaker force. The sap extracted in an earth bowl, exposed to sunlight first as it were, and the remaining juice stored.

obols: An obol or *obolus* was a small Greek coin, which gave its name to a small weight used by ancient and medieval apothecaries. Six obols made a drachma.

albugo: White opacity of the cornea.

III.11. Water Germander

Water germander grows in hilly and marshy places; its leaves are like those of wall germander, larger but not so deeply crenated around their margins; it is like garlic to the sense of smell, but **binding** and rather bitter to the taste; the small stalks are square, from which grows a reddish flower.

binding: Meaning astringent here.

The herb possesses a warming property; diuretic when it is green, pounded, and given in a drink; and dried but soaked in wine for snakebites and poisons, for gnawing pains of the stomach, and dysentery and difficult **micturition**; 2 **drachmas** of weight with **hydromel**. It cleans out also a thick purulence from the chest, and it is useful too for cough of long standing, and lesions and convulsions, mixed in a lozenge with garden cress and honey and dried resin; and having been made into a wax-salve it soothes an abdomen long inflamed. And it is also useful for gout smeared on with strong vinegar or being laid on with water; when applied as a pessary it causes menstruation; it closes up wounds and cleans out sores of long standing and when mixed with honey, it promotes healing; dried, it retards overgrowths of flesh. But also the juice is drunk for "the troubles" as they have been called; the most efficacious is the Pontic and the Cretan.

micturition: Urination.

drachmas: A drachma was an ancient Greek currency (still used in Greece until 2001), which gave its name to a weight used by ancient and medieval apothecaries. A drachma was composed of six obols.

hydromel: A mixture of honey and water commonly used in ancient and medieval medicine.

DOCUMENT 24:
Galen, the Boastful Practitioner: *On the Affected Places*[9]

> In this passage from his treatise *On the Affected Places* Galen (ca. 130–210 CE) boasts of his seemingly magical skills in the diagnosis and prognosis of difficult diseases, knitting together obscure clues into a satisfying medical narrative. As a trained philosopher, he used logic in the process now known as "differential diagnosis" to define and distinguish the patient's symptoms precisely and thereby identify the ailment and its cause, make a prognosis, and propose a suitable treatment.

ℰ

When I came to Rome for the first time I was greatly admired by the philosopher Glaucon on account of a similar diagnosis. Finding me on the road, he said to me that I had arrived opportunely; then taking my hand, he said: "We are quite near an invalid whom I have seen just now, and I wish you would come to visit him with me. He is a Sicilian physician whom you have seen a few days ago walking with me." "What is the cause of his illness?" I said. Placing himself at my side, he said very frankly and plainly—for he was not one to cheat or play tricks—"Gorgias and Apelas informed me yesterday that you have made diagnoses and prognoses which approach to divination rather than to the art of medicine. I desire, then, to have a proof, not of your knowledge, but of the power of the art of medicine, and to ascertain if it can furnish such an astonishing diagnosis and prognosis."

During this conversation we had arrived at the door of the patient, so that I had not been able to reply to his request, nor to tell him, what you know I often repeat, that sometimes there are, fortunate for us, indubitable signs, but that sometimes everything is doubtful, and that consequently we have to await the results of a second or third examination. At the outer gate we met a domestic who was carrying from the sick room to the dunghill a vessel containing excrements resembling the washings of flesh—that is to say, thin and bloody fluid, a constant sign of an affection of the liver. Without appearing to have noticed anything, I went with Glaucon to the physician, and I was putting my hand to his arm, wishing to know if there was inflammation of the organ or simply **atony**. The patient, who was himself a physician, as I have mentioned, said that he had just returned to bed after having been at stool. "Consider, therefore," he added, "that the frequency of the pulse is increased by the effort I have made in rising." Thus

atony: A condition in which a muscle has lost all its strength, often associated with uterine or gastrointestinal conditions.

---

9   James Finlayson, *Galen: A Bibliographical Demonstration in the Library of the Faculty of Physicians and Surgeons of Glasgow, December 9th, 1891* (British Medical Association, 1892), 11–12.

he spoke, and as for me, I ascertained in the pulse the sign of inflammation. Then, seeing placed at the window a pot containing hyssop prepared with honey-coloured water, I bethought me that the physician believed himself affected with a pleurisy, on account of feeling at the false ribs the pain which sometimes also appears there in inflammation of the liver. I thought that, as he experienced this pain, his respiration was frequent and small, and that he was tormented with short paroxysms of cough; in a word, he believed himself affected with pleurisy, and so had made a preparation of hyssop and honey water. Recognising, then, that good fortune had given me the means of raising myself in the estimation of Glaucon, I placed my hand on the false ribs on the right side of the patient, and indicating the place, I said that he suffered in this region. The patient confessed it, and Glaucon, believing that the pulse alone had sufficed for this diagnosis of the affected place, showed visible signs of admiration. To astonish him further, I added, "If you have admitted that you suffer there, acknowledge also that you experience the necessity of coughing, and that at pretty long intervals you are seized with a short, dry cough, without expectoration." As I said these words he coughed, by chance, exactly in the way I had indicated. Then Glaucon, astonished, and being unable to contain himself, heaped on me well-earned praise, with a loud voice. "Do not suppose," said I, "that these are the only things which art can divine regarding patients; there are others which I will mention. The patient himself will be my witness." Then addressing him: "When you breathe more deeply, you feel a sharper pain at the place which I have marked; you experience also weight in the right **hypochonder**." At these words the patient could not restrain himself; full of admiration he joined his exclamations to those of Glaucon. Recognising the success which I had obtained on this occasion, I wished to risk a word about the twinges at the clavicle; but although knowing well that this accompanies grave inflammation of the liver, as **scirrhus**, I did not dare to advance this, fearing to compromise the praises which they had lavished on me. I had the idea of sliding in this remark, with precaution, and turning to the patient I said: "Shortly, you will experience twinges at the clavicle, if you have not already felt them." He confessed this to be the fact; and I said, looking at the patient, who was struck with astonishment, "I will not add further to my indications than this divination; I will announce the opinion which the patient himself has formed of the disease with which he has been affected."

Glaucon said that he did not any longer despair of this divination; and the patient, stupefied by this singular promise, gave me a piercing glance, and close attention to my words. When I had told him that he believed himself affected with a pleurisy, he acknowledged the fact, testifying his admiration; and not he only but also the servant who came to make the affusions of oil as if had a pleurisy. Glaucon since this time conceived a high

hypochonder: More commonly hypochondrium, the upper area of the abdomen, around the lower ribs.

scirrhus: Hardening of a gland or organ.

opinion of me and of the medical art, which he had esteemed but slightly before, never having found himself associated with remarkable men who were consummate masters of the art.

DOCUMENT 25:

Galen, *On Black Bile*: Praising and Rewriting Hippocrates[10]

Black bile was the most difficult of the four Hippocratic humors to identify
and analyze: it was credited with causing the worst of diseases but it did not
seem to match with a specific bodily fluid like blood, phlegm, or yellow bile.
Galen (ca. 130–210 CE) therefore wrote an entire treatise, *On Black Bile*, to
determine what Hippocrates supposedly said about the subject and then build
on that with his own ideas. He starts in his usual fashion by condemning
earlier authors on the subject of black bile, while praising Hippocrates and
quoting from his *Nature of Man* (Document 7, pp. 29–32) and *Aphorisms*
(Document 10, pp. 39–44). He then gives a lengthy explanation, based on his
own experience, of how to distinguish black bile from dried blood and other
dark or black substances in the human body.

ల

The variability of blood both in color and in consistency therefore demonstrates that all the humors are contained together in the veins and arteries.
But this is also abundantly clear from what has already been said, and
especially from those things, which are found written by Hippocrates in
the book **On the Nature of Man**. I have treated these statements at great
length in my work *On Elements*. But it is now necessary to bring before us
one of those subjects, so let us begin with that passage where [Hippocrates]
writes the following:

> *On the Nature of Man*: See this Hippocratic text above in Document 7, pp. 29–32.

[Galen reproduces here a lengthy quote about the four humors from the
Hippocratic text *Nature of Man*, found above in Document 7, paragraph IV,
p. 29.]

Therefore no one who is versed in the medical arts can deny that
Hippocrates has spoken the truth here, namely, that an ensouled body is
healthy when the humors have obtained a balance of temperament, but
that it grows sick either when there is an excess of any of those humors in
the whole body (that is, in all its hollow places) or when this occurs in any
single part of the body. For when I had discussed, a little while ago, those
diseases that occur in a single part of the body because of black bile, I also
declared that some people are filled with **melancholy** after the removal of
varicose veins or hemorrhoids. It is therefore consistent with reason that

> **melancholy:** Black bile (*melancholia*) and any disease engendered by that humor, which often produces sad feelings, hence the modern "melancholy."

---

10 Galen, *De atra bile*, in *Claudii Galeni Opera Omnia*, Vol. V, edited by Karl Kühn (Leipzig, 1823),
119–22, 126–28, 130–31, 144. Original translation by the author of this volume.

conditions are produced in parts of the body hidden deep inside similar to those which are found on the skin. For surely, according to that reasoning, if yellow bile should remain long in any one part of the body, **erysipelas** will be generated, but if black bile, carbuncles and **cancer**. To be sure, the parts that are deep within the body in no way possess an unchanging constitution, but they also are subject to the same diseases.

In these statements it is therefore possible for us to recognize the efficient cause with certainty: first yellow bile and then black bile are clearly evident in these cases. They gnaw at each other variously in the internal organs (that is to say, in whatsoever part they more firmly adhere) and sometimes bring about an entirely incurable dysentery. On this subject Hippocrates wrote in his *Aphorisms*, "Dysentery is lethal if it arises from black bile."

... I do not intend in any way to explain the faculties of the other humors, for I had, admittedly, proposed to treat only black bile, the generation of which Hippocrates claims is absolutely necessary. But having said this, he taught how it might not be generated in excess, beginning from evident signs. For black bile often appears to be produced both in those ensouled bodies, which are hotter and drier in temperament, as well as during hotter and drier times of the year, regions, and constitutions, as well as in those ways of life, which are subject to excess labor, worry, and sleeplessness, not to mention in excessively dry and heavy foods. In fact, the color of the whole body is blacker in those people who are naturally suited to accumulate this sort of bile, as well as in those burning diseases, which have their origin beyond moisture. In these cases the black bile flows whenever blood bursts forth or drips slowly.

Therefore these evidential signs indicate the causes by which black bile is produced. But concerning the purgation of black bile, these evidential signs will also show a path to understanding. When the spleen is badly diseased, either from inflammation, from hardening of the tissue, or from weakness, it provokes a change toward a darker, infected color throughout the whole body. But black bile is always darker in the liver, and especially in animals of hotter and drier temperament, such as those with sharp teeth, just as conversely those animals possessed of a colder and moister temperament are not so black in the spleen, like pigs.... Persuaded by these signs, the most eminent of ancient physicians and philosophers claimed that the liver was purged by the spleen, that is, when it drew out all the filth from the blood, that sort of material which appeared, as it is said, like the dregs of wine or the waste from pressing olives. But the younger physicians, who prefer to establish medical sects, just as they have spoken falsely about many things, so also they claim that a doctor has no need for the observation of humors in his medical practice, and that, above all else, purgative drugs are pointlessly called "purgative." For they say that these drugs equally purge all the humors that are found in the body, and not just those which seem to cause harm.

But Hippocrates, assuming that those drugs purge something, as agreed, demonstrated that the four humors were contained in the human body for the entire span of life, nor was there any age, nor time of year, nor bodily disposition in which they were not all present. From the following facts—that the drugs attracting yellow bile are of benefit to those suffering from the "**royal disease**," while those which are called *hydragoga*, that is, "leading out water," clear up the dropsy which is called *ascites* because of the similarity of the two, and those drugs which remove black bile prevent **elephantiasis** and cancer from growing—it seemed evident enough to the ancient physicians that each of the purgative drugs attracts its own appropriate humor.

... Hippocrates therefore seems to have been an honorable and upstanding sort of man, a lover neither of ambition nor glory, but only of truth. But if someone claims that he pursued glory or honor for its own sake, it certainly would have been very easy for such a man to gain them, if only he wished to contend in writing with the more established and older medical sects, even if one were not then very illustrious. In truth, those who followed after him claimed, with insatiable desire, an undeserved reputation, they established their own depraved sects and afterwards put forth arguments against those physicians older than them, although some of them were gifted with honorable morals and elegant speech, among whom some might also number **Erasistratus**. But the war against Hippocrates forced even Erasistratus to write in defense of himself.

... In this respect, I will now add what I have firmly learned about black bile through long experience, which surely will be of use to those who eagerly pursue the actual work of medicine and not merely sophistic arguments about it. Concerning all the diseases which are caused by the humor black bile, if you immediately and powerfully purge using the drugs that evacuate this humor, in such a way you will prevent them from increasing to the point of cancer.

royal disease: An ancient euphemism for jaundice (not to be confused with hemophilia, which is now sometimes called the "royal disease").

elephantiasis: Most likely leprosy, now known as Hansen's Disease, but the term could apply to any number of conditions that cause extreme swelling of the limbs or very rough skin.

Erasistratus: A Hellenistic physician and anatomist, ca. 304–250 BCE. He came from Seleucid Syria but moved to Alexandria where, according to tradition, he founded a school of anatomy. He and his contemporary physician Herophilus (335–280 BCE) made some of the most important contributions to ancient anatomy, including the identification of veins and arteries, by dissecting cadavers and perhaps even living patients.

DOCUMENT 26:
Herodian on a Plague in the Roman Empire[11]

> The Roman historian Herodian of Antioch (ca. 170–240 CE) describes
> in his *History of the Roman Empire since the Death of Marcus Aurelius* how
> Commodus, co-emperor with his father Marcus Aurelius for the years
> 177–180 CE, avoided getting sick during the so-called Antonine Plague of
> ca. 165–180 CE (perhaps smallpox or measles). The Roman doctors prescribed
> sweet smells and perfumes to block the polluted air that was believed to
> spread the plague.

e

About this time, plague struck all Italy. The suffering was especially severe
in Rome, since the city, which received people from all over the world, was
overcrowded. The city suffered great loss of both men and animals. Then,
on the advice of his physicians, Commodus left Rome for Laurentum. This
region enjoyed the shade from extensive laurel groves (whence the area
derives its name); it was cooler there and seemed to be a safe haven. The
emperor is said to have counteracted the pollution in the air by the fragrant
scent of the laurels and the refreshing shade of the trees. At the direction
of their doctors, those who remained in Rome filled their nostrils and ears
with fragrant oils and used perfume and incense constantly, for some said
that the sweet odor, entering first, filled up the sensory passages and kept out
the poison in the air; or, if any poison should enter, it would be neutralized
by the stronger odors. The plague, however, continued to rage unchecked for
a long time, and many men died, as well as domestic animals of all kinds.

---

11   Herodian of Antioch, *History of the Roman Empire since the Death of Marcus Aurelius*, translated by
     Edward C. Echols (Berkeley, 1961), 1.12.1–2.

PART 4

Practical Medicine for the Roman Family and Home (ca. 1–500 CE)

Not all the learned doctors in the Roman Republic or Empire were Greek. Some Latin authors addressed medical issues, but they nonetheless support the infamous summary of ancient history, "The Greeks had good brains, the Romans had good drains." That is to say, we know the Greeks primarily for their philosophy, science, and literature, while we know the Romans for their impressive cities, roads, and aqueducts. When we find Romans applying medical theory, they often did so for the purposes of infrastructure, or estate and military management. For example, the Roman author Marcus Terentius Varro (116–27 BCE) describes in his work *De re rustica* (*On Agriculture*, Document 27) the proper location of an estate so that the air and water are most healthful for the inhabitants. The work is written in the classical form of a dialogue, and this passage is spoken by a visiting expert on agriculture, Gnaeus Tremelius Scrofa, visiting the estate of one Gaius Fundanius, Varro's father-in-law. Varro's exploration of the causes of disease on landed estates leads him to explore the possibility that minute creatures (*animalculae*) could be the cause of certain diseases. Similarly, the late Roman author Vegetius (ca. 400 CE) wrote a work, *De re militari* (*On the Military*, Document 28) concerning the training and maintenance of the military, in which he addresses the health of the troops. Vegetius's recommendations seem to draw on both real experiences from the field as well as medical treatises like the Hippocratic work *Airs, Waters, Places* (Document 11, pp. 42–45).

In most, but not all ancient written accounts of healing, the physician is male. However, it is likely that women practiced a great deal of informal medicine and served as professional midwives in ancient Mediterranean cultures. There are records of a small number of women working as physicians, though classical scholars debate how common they were and what forms of healing they practiced.[1] Women are also the focus, of course, in

---

[1]   See Holt N. Parker, "Women Doctors in Greece, Rome, and the Byzantine Empire," in *Women Healers and Physicians: Climbing a Long Hill*, edited by Lilian R. Furst (UP of Kentucky, 1997), 131–50.

writings about childbirth and gynecology. The woman Agnodike is described in a number of sources, including the *Fables* (Document 29) of the Roman author Hyginus (d. 17 CE), as the founder of obstetrics. Though she is most likely fictional, the story nonetheless demonstrates Hellenistic and Roman attitudes toward women and professional medical care.

Despite the legend of Agnodike and the dominance of women in the field of obstetrics, the author of the most popular ancient work on the topic was male. Soranus of Ephesus was a Greek physician active in Rome during the reigns of emperor Trajan and Hadrian in the early second century CE. His *Gynaikeia* (*Gynecology*) is a manual for midwives or for those seeking a good midwife. In Document 30, Soranus describes the care of a newly pregnant woman according to **Methodist** medical principles. Soranus also wrote *On Acute and Chronic Diseases*, which survives in a Latin translation by Caelius Aurelianus in the fifth century CE. His *Gynecology* was translated into Latin in the sixth century in an adaptation called *Gynaecia* by one Muscio, which represented learned gynecology for medieval Europe until the twelfth century. It was primarily through Muscio's work that medieval Europeans knew about Soranus of Ephesus.[2]

Roman medicine drew much of its theory from Greek philosophical medicine but often remained based essentially on traditional agriculture, life at home, and domestic religious practices.[3] The modified Hippocratic medicine of Galen was only for the elites and the emperor. Much actual healing among the Romans was simple, homely, and eminently practical. This can be seen clearly in Cato the Elder's description of Roman medical remedies in his treatise *De Agricultura* (ca. 160 BCE, Document 31), in which cures are made from Roman household ingredients like wine, ham, or cabbage. Cato also employs magical charms without distinguishing natural from supernatural remedies.

Pliny the Elder (23–79 CE) is ancient Rome's most famous naturalist, thanks to his encyclopedia in 37 volumes, the *Natural History*. He includes many medicinal remedies in his sections on plants, animals, and stones. For both Cato and Pliny, Roman medicine is not a theory or school of thought, but a collection of recipes passed down the generations and protected by the *paterfamilias* as head of his household. The connection between medicine and other household affairs is clearly demonstrated in Document 32, where Pliny describes medical remedies made from wool. Pliny died in the eruption of Mount Vesuvius in 79 CE, apparently while trying to rescue his family by ship. Later in the Roman imperial era, the physician Quintus Serenus

Methodist: An ancient medical school or "sect." See Document 19, pp. 69–70, for a description of their beliefs.

---

2   Ann Ellis Hanson and Monica H. Green, "Soranus of Ephesus: *Methodicorum princeps*," in *Aufstieg und Niedergang der römischen Welt*, II, 37.2, edited by W. Haase and H. Temporini (1994), 968–1075.

3   Scarborough, *Roman Medicine*, 15.

(second or third century CE) made a brief compendium called the *Liber Medicinalis* (Document 33), in which he put medical remedies and information into Latin verse. Both Cato and Quintus Serenus prescribe natural remedies along with magical spells: the former records magical charms to be said over a dislocated limb and the latter provides the earliest known example of the magic word ABRACADABRA as part of a cure for a fever.

DOCUMENT 27:

Varro, *De re rustica*: An Early Germ Theory?[4]

In his work *De re rustica* (*On Agriculture*) Marcus Terentius Varro (116–27 BCE) describes the proper location of an estate so that the air and water are most healthful for the inhabitants. Varro suggests the possibility that minute creatures (*animalculae*) could be the cause of certain diseases.

ℰ

"When you plan to build, try your best to locate the steading at the foot of a wooded hill where the pastures are rich, and turn it so as to catch the healthiest prevailing breeze. The best situation is facing the east so to secure shade in summer and sun in winter. But if you must build on the bank of a river, take care that you do not let the steading face the river, for it will be very cold in winter and unhealthy in summer. Like precautions must be taken against swampy places for the same reasons and particularly because as they dry, swamps breed certain ***animalculae*** which cannot be seen with the eyes and which we breathe through the nose and mouth into the body where they cause grave maladies."

"But," said Fundanius, "suppose I inherited a farm like that, what should I do to avoid the malady you describe?"

"The answer to that question is easy," said Agrius. "You should sell the farm for what you can get for it: and if you can't sell it, give it away."

Scrofa resumed: "Take care to avoid having the steading face the direction from which disagreeable winds blow, yet you should not build in a hollow. High ground is the best location for a steading: for by ventilation all noxious gases are dissipated, and the steading is healthier if exposed to the sun all day: with the further advantage that any insects which may be bred in or brought upon the premises are either blown away or quickly perish where there is no damp. Sudden rains and overflowed streams are dangerous to those who have their steadings in low or hollow places, and they are more at the hazard of the ruthless hand of the robber because he is able to take advantage of those who are unprepared. Against either of these risks the higher places are safer."

animalculae: A Latin word meaning "tiny animals," which Varro probably used simply to mean small insects like gnats or mosquitoes, but in later centuries it would be used by scientists to describe the first minute organisms seen under microscopes.

---

4   Varro, *De re rustica* I.12, in *Roman Farm Management. The Treatises of Cato and Varro Done into English* ..., translated by F.H. Belvoir (New York, 1913), 94–96.

Vegetius, *De re militari*: Preserving the Health of Imperial Troops[5]

> The late Roman author Vegetius (ca. 400 CE) wrote *De re militari* (*On the Military*) about the training and maintenance of the military, including the health of the troops. His recommendations seem to draw on both field experience and medical treatises like the Hippocratic *Airs, Waters, Places* (Document 11, pp. 42–45). *De re militari* remained one of the most important military manuals through the entire Middle Ages.

e

Means of Preserving It in Health

The next article is of the greatest importance: the means of preserving the health of the troops. This depends on the choice of situation and water, on the season of the year, medicine, and exercise. As to the situation, the army should never continue in the neighborhood of unwholesome marshes any length of time, or on dry plains or eminences without some sort of shade or shelter. In the summer, the troops should never encamp without tents. And their marches, in that season of the year when the heat is excessive, should begin by break of day so that they may arrive at the place of destination in good time. Otherwise they will contract diseases from the heat of the weather and the fatigue of the march. In severe winter they should never march in the night in frost and snow, or be exposed to want of wood or clothes. A soldier, starved with cold, can neither be healthy nor fit for service. The water must be wholesome and not marshy. Bad water is a kind of poison and the cause of epidemic distempers.

It is the duty of the officers of the legion, of the tribunes, and even of the commander-in-chief himself, to take care that the sick soldiers are supplied with proper diet and diligently attended by the physicians. For little can be expected from men who have both the enemy and diseases to struggle with. However, the best judges of the service have always been of the opinion that daily practice of the military exercises is much more efficacious towards the health of an army than all the art of medicine. For this reason they exercised their infantry without intermission. If it rained or snowed, they performed under cover; and if fine weather, in the field. They also were assiduous in exercising their cavalry, not only in plains, but also on uneven ground, broken and cut with ditches. The horses as well as the men were

---

5   Vegetius, *De re militari* III.2, in *Military Institutions of Vegetius in Five Books*, translated by John Clarke (London, 1767).

thus trained, both on the above mentioned account and to prepare them for action. Hence we may perceive the importance and necessity of a strict observance of the military exercises in an army, since health in the camp and victory in the field depend on them. If a numerous army continues long in one place in the summer or in the autumn, the waters become corrupt and the air infected. Malignant and fatal distempers proceed from this and can be avoided only by frequent changes of encampments.

DOCUMENT 29:

The Legend of Agnodike, a Greek Midwife and Physician[6]

The legendary midwife Agnodike is described in the *Fables* of the Roman author Hyginus (d. 17 CE) as the founder of obstetrics. Her story and the creation of professional midwifery is placed in the context of the distant Athenian past, when supposedly only men could perform any sort of medical care. This probably does not represent a historical reality but rather the common desire among classical authors to identify a specific origin story for their customs, crafts, and careers.

℮

The ancients did not have midwives, and for this reason women died of shame,[7] since the Athenians were afraid that any servant or woman might learn the art of medicine. Because of this, a virgin girl named Agnodike desired to learn medicine. Pursuing her desire, she cut off her hair, put on men's clothing, and presented herself to a certain man named Herophilus for an education. When she had learned this art and heard a woman in labor, she came to her. And when this woman did not want to believe her, reckoning she was a man, Agnodike lifted her tunic and showed her that she was a woman. In such a way she began to cure women. When the male physicians perceived that they were not allowed to treat women, they began to make accusations against Agnodike, saying she was a beardless slave boy and a corruptor of the women, who were only pretending sickness. And when the **Areopagites** sat in judgment, they began to condemn Agnodike. Agnodike lifted her tunic before them and showed that she was a woman. Then the male physicians began to accuse her more vehemently. Because of this the noble women came before the court and said, you are not our husbands, but rather enemies, because you condemn the woman who discovered health for us. After that the Athenians changed the law so that freeborn women could study medicine.

Areopagites: An Athenian council of elders, named for their seat on the Areopagus, a hill near the Acropolis in Athens.

---

6   *Hygini Fabulae* no. 274, edited by M. Schmidt (Jena, 1872), 149–50. Original translation by the editor of this volume.

7   What is implied here is that a good Greek woman would never reveal her body to a male physician.

DOCUMENT 30:

Soranus of Ephesus: Instructions for Midwives[8]

Soranus of Ephesus (second century CE) wrote his book *Gynecology* as a manual for midwives or for those seeking a good midwife. In this passage, Soranus describes the care needed to preserve the implantation of the "seed" (in modern biology, this means the fertilized embryo and not the male semen) in a newly pregnant woman. The passage demonstrates contemporary Greco-Roman thought on pregnancy, women, and Methodist medical principles.

ℰ

What Care Should Be Given to Pregnant Women?

The care of pregnant women has three stages. For the care during the first period is aimed at the preservation of the injected seed; during the second, at the alleviation of subsequent symptoms, such as the treatment of the **pica** which ensues; during the last period which is already close to parturition, it aims at the perfection of the embryo and a ready endurance of parturition. Of these, we shall at present make inquiry into the first.

When conception has taken place, one must beware of every excess and change both bodily and psychic. For the seed is evacuated through fright, sorrow, sudden joy and, generally, by severe mental upset; through vigorous exercise, forced detention of the breath, coughing, sneezing, blows, and falls, especially those on the hips; by lifting heavy weights, leaping, sitting on hard sedan chairs, by the administration of drugs, by the application of pungent substances and **sternutatives**; through want, indigestion, drunkenness, vomiting, diarrhea; by a flow of blood from the nose, from hemorrhoids or other places; through relaxation due to some heating agent, through marked fever, rigors, cramps and, in general, everything inducing a forcible movement by which a miscarriage may be produced. Now of these things, those within our control ought to be eschewed, and one ought to keep the woman who has conceived quietly in bed for one or two days when she should use anointments in a simple fashion in order to strengthen her appetite as well as to aid the assimilation of food offered her. But at the same time she should not allow massage of the abdomen lest through the associated movement in that region the attaching seed be torn off.

One ought to anoint her with freshly extracted oil from unripe olives and should give her less food and that of the cereal type. One ought to

pica: Craving non-food substances like dirt or chalk, common among small children, but often associated with women during pregnancy or after childbirth.

sternutatives: Substances that cause sneezing.

---

8   Soranus, *Gynecology* I.xiv, translated by Owsei Temkin, with Nicholson J. Eastman, Ludwig Edelstein, and Alan F. Guttmacher (Baltimore, 1956), 45–47.

omit the bath, if possible, for seven days; for the bath, belonging to those things which loosen the texture of the whole body, will also help to enfeeble the delicate structure of the seed. Otherwise one would have to assume that wounds not yet safely united are further widened by a bath and the extremely compact bodies of athletes are relaxed, yet on the other hand, the seed will not melt away when its structure is still soft and has only just become solid. Hence there is nothing strange in the rejection of wine too for an equal number of days, so that the distribution of food may not become violent and overpowering. For just as the parts of broken bones, if not moved, become fused, so the seed too becomes implanted securely and firmly in the uterus, if not shaken by moving agents. On the other hand, to be sure, one must not continue this treatment for a longer period lest, the body becoming exhausted by the deprivation of wine and food, the uterus become languid together with it; rather one ought to change it little by little. As early as the second day, she ought to take passive exercise in a stool or a large sedan chair (for being drawn by animals is to be rejected since it shakes violently); then she ought to take a short, easy walk in leisurely fashion lengthening it with every day; and she ought to partake of foods of neutral character, such as fish which are not greasy, meats which are not very fat, and vegetables which are not pungent. But she should avoid everything pungent, such as garlic, onions, leeks, preserved meat or fish, and very moist foods; for the latter are apt to disintegrate, while pungent substances cause flatulence and besides are **solvent and attenuating**, and hence we approve of them in chronic patients for the removal of **callosities** for instance. But it is absolutely illogical not to realize that things which irritate, attenuate, and wear down the whole physique, and which dissolve callosities, that all these things, apportioned by distribution to the various parts of the uterus, will soften the seed much more, which is like mucus as long as it is not yet held together by coagulation. And she must also beware of intercourse; for it too causes movement in the whole body in general and especially in the various parts about the uterus which need rest. For just as the stomach when quiet retains the food, but when shaken often ejects through vomiting what it has received, so also the uterus when not shaken holds fast the seed; when agitated, however, discharges it.

She should take fairly warm baths for the sake of both the air and the water, without prolonged and copious sweating lest the body become enfeebled and lose its tone. And the cold bath ought to be used in moderation too, so that no shivering sensation may arise. And after the rubdown she must fast until the body has become quiet and the disturbance of the breath and the agitation of the body fluids have calmed down. Later, for a fairly long period, she ought to drink water before meals or, if accustomed to it, a little weak wine.

solvent and attenuating: Substances that dissolve and thin out hardenings or excess fluids in the body, according to premodern medical theories.

callosities: Hardenings of the skin, calluses.

DOCUMENT 31:

Cato the Elder's Roman Remedies: Cabbage, Wine, and Magic[9]

> Roman medicine, although based partly on Greek philosophical medicine, remained homely and practical in its ingredients and methods. This can be seen in Cato the Elder's description of native Roman medical remedies in his treatise *De Agricultura* (ca. 160 BCE). Most of Cato's cures are made with ingredients found in any Roman household, like wine, ham, or his favorite vegetable, cabbage. Notes are not given below for the many Roman measures Cato uses: *congius, hemina, mina*, drachm, sextarius, etc.

ᴇ𝓋

126. For gripes, for loose bowels, for tapeworms and stomach-worms, if troublesome: Take 30 acid pomegranates, crush, place in a jar with 3 *congii* of strong black wine, and seal the vessel. Thirty days later open and use. Drink a *hemina* before eating.

dyspepsia: Indigestion.

strangury: Difficulty urinating or painful urination due to a blockage in the bladder.

127. Remedy for **dyspepsia** and **strangury**: Gather pomegranate blossoms when they open, and place 3 *minae* of them in an amphora. Add one quadrantal of old wine and a mina of clean crushed root of fennel; seal the vessel and thirty days later open and use. You may drink this as freely as you wish without risk, when you wish to digest your food and to urinate. The same wine will clear out tapeworms and stomach-worms if it is blended in this way. Bid the patient refrain from eating in the evening, and the next morning macerate 1 drachm of pulverized incense, 1 drachm of boiled honey, and a sextarius of wine of wild marjoram. Administer to him before he eats, and, for a child, according to age, a triobolus and a *hemina*. Have him climb a pillar and jump down ten times, and walk about....

156. Of the medicinal value of the cabbage: It is the cabbage which surpasses all other vegetables. It may be eaten either cooked or raw; if you eat it raw, dip it into vinegar. It promotes digestion marvellously and is an excellent laxative, and the urine is wholesome for everything. If you wish to drink deep at a banquet and to enjoy your dinner, eat as much raw cabbage as you wish, seasoned with vinegar, before dinner, and likewise after dinner eat some half a dozen leaves; it will make you feel as if you had not dined, and you can drink as much as you please....

---

9   Cato and Varro, *On Agriculture*, translated by W.D. Hooper and H.B. Ash (Harvard UP, 1934), 126–27, 156, 158–60.

158. Recipe for a purgative, if you wish to purge thoroughly: Take a pot and pour into it six *sextarii* of water and add the hock of a ham, or, if you have no hock, a half-pound of ham-scraps with as little fat as possible. Just as it comes to a boil, add two cabbage leaves, two beet plants with the roots, a shoot of fern, a bit of the **mercury-plant**, two pounds of mussels, a capito fish and one scorpion, six snails, and a handful of lentils. Boil all together down to three *sextarii* of liquid, without adding oil. Take one *sextarius* of this while warm, add one *cyathus* of Coan wine, drink, and rest. Take a second and a third dose in the same way, and you will be well purged. You may drink diluted Coan wine in addition, if you wish. Any one of the many ingredients mentioned above is sufficient to move the bowels; but there are so many ingredients in this concoction that it is an excellent purgative, and, besides, it is agreeable.

mercury-plant: A member of the genus *Mercurialis* in the spurge family, probably herb mercury (*Mercurialis annua*).

159. To prevent chafing: When you set out on a journey, keep a small branch of Pontic wormwood under the anus.

160. Any kind of dislocation may be cured by the following charm: Take a green reed four or five feet long and split it down the middle, and let two men hold it to your hips. Begin to chant: ***motas uaeta daries dardares astataries dissunapiter*** and continue until they meet. Brandish a knife over them, and when the reeds meet so that one touches the other, grasp with the hand and cut right and left. If the pieces are applied to the dislocation or the fracture, it will heal. And none the less chant every day, and, in the case of a dislocation, in this manner, if you wish: ***huat haut haut istasis tarsis ardannabou dannaustra***.

motas uaeta … dannaustra: The italicized phrases in paragraph 160 are nonsense but some individual words come from Archaic Latin. By Cato's time, they had lost their meaning (if they ever had one) but retained a magical power that was believed to be transmitted through chanting them along with symbols of healing, like the knife.

DOCUMENT 32:
Pliny the Elder's Homespun Medicine: Remedies Derived from Wool[10]

The Roman encyclopedist Pliny the Elder (23–79 CE) included many medicinal remedies in the sections on plants, animals, and stones in his *Natural History*, such as the description below of the uses of wool and eggs in healing. The items and methods described here are probably closer to daily Roman medical practice than the herbs and spices described in the *De materia medica* of Dioscorides (Document 23, pp. 78–79).

୧ଂ

I shall begin then with some remedies that are well known, those namely, which are derived from wool and from the eggs of birds, thus giving due honour to those substances which hold the principal place in the estimation of mankind; though at the same time I shall be necessitated to speak of some others out of their proper place, according as occasion may offer. I should not have been at a loss for high-flown language with which to grace my narrative, had I made it my design to regard anything else than what, as being strictly trustworthy, becomes my work: for among the very first remedies mentioned, we find those said to be derived from the ashes and nest of the phoenix, as though, forsooth, its existence were a well ascertained fact, and not altogether a fable. And then besides, it would be a mere mockery to describe remedies that can only return to us once in a thousand years.

The ancient Romans attributed to wool a degree of religious importance even, and it was in this spirit that they enjoined that the bride should touch the door-posts of her husband's house with wool. In addition to dress and protection from the cold, wool, in an unwashed state, used in combination with oil, and wine or vinegar, supplies us with numerous remedies, according as we stand in need of an emollient or an excitant, an astringent or a laxative. Wetted from time to time with these liquids, greasy wool is applied to sprained limbs, and to sinews that are suffering from pain. In the case of sprains, some persons are in the habit of adding salt, while others, again, apply pounded rue and grease, in wool: the same, too, in the case of contusions or tumours. Wool will improve the breath, it is said, if the teeth and gums are rubbed with it, mixed with honey; it is very good, too, for **phrenitis**, used as a fumigation. To arrest bleeding at the nose, wool is introduced into the nostrils with oil of roses; or it is used in another manner, the ears being well plugged with it. In the case of inveterate ulcers it is applied topically

phrenitis: An inflammation of the brain that was believed to produce "frenzy" (*phrenesis*).

---

10 Pliny the Elder, *The Natural History*, translated by John Bostock (Taylor and Francis, 1855).

with honey: soaked in wine or vinegar, or in cold water and oil, and then squeezed out, it is used for the cure of wounds.

Rams' wool, washed in cold water, and steeped in oil, is used for female complaints, and to allay inflammations of the uterus. **Procidence** of the uterus is reduced by using this wool in the form of a fumigation. Greasy wool, used as a plaster and as a pessary, brings away the dead fetus, and arrests uterine discharges. Bites inflicted by a mad dog are plugged with unwashed wool, the application being removed at the end of seven days. Applied with cold water, it is a cure for **agnails**: steeped in a mixture of boiling nitre, sulphur, oil, vinegar, and tar, and applied twice a day, as warm as possible, it allays pains in the loins. By making ligatures with unwashed rams' wool about the extremities of the limbs, bleeding is effectually stopped.

In all cases, the wool most esteemed is that from the neck of the animal; the best kinds of wool being those of Galatia, Tarentum, Attica, and Miletus. For excoriations, blows, bruises, contusions, crushes, galls, falls, pains in the head and other parts, and for inflammation of the stomach, unwashed wool is applied, with a mixture of vinegar and oil of roses. Reduced to ashes, it is applied to contusions, wounds, and burns, and forms an ingredient in ophthalmic compositions. It is employed, also, for fistulas and suppurations of the ears. For this last purpose, some persons take the wool as it is shorn, while others pluck it from the fleece; they then cut off the ends of it, and after drying and carding it, lay it in pots of unbaked earth, steep it well in honey, and burn it. Others, again, arrange it in layers alternately with chips of torchpine, and, after sprinkling it with oil, set fire to it: they then rub the ashes into small vessels with the hands, and let them settle in water there. This operation is repeated and the water changed several times, until at last the ashes are found to be slightly astringent, without the slightest pungency; upon which, they are put by for use, being possessed of certain caustic properties, and extremely useful as a detergent for the eyelids.

Procidence: When the uterus starts to fall out of the vagina; now usually called prolapse.

agnails: An archaic English variant of hangnails.

DOCUMENT 33:
Popular Medicine in Verse: The *Liber medicinalis*[11]

The Roman imperial physician Quintus Serenus made a brief medical compendium called the *Liber medicinalis*, perhaps in the third century CE, in which he put medical remedies and information into Latin verse. This helped with learning and memorization, and the work circulated widely in the Middle Ages. This work, like those of Cato and Pliny (Documents 31 and 32), show how Roman imperial medicine mingled technical Greek medical theory, home remedies, and magical charms (including the earliest example of "ABRACADABRA") into a new and vibrant medical system.

ᴇ

Curing a Tertian Fever

There is also a fever reviving on alternate days:
It divides time like the weight of an even scale.
Therefore, so you can halt such a burning,
Fold cumin grains, without their tails, into wax,
Put this in a red leather skin and bind it to the patient's neck.
A branch of pennyroyal, veiled with a cloak of wool,
Will offer healing odors at the expected time of fever.
Moreover, a smashed bug should be swallowed with an egg:
This is horrible to touch, but tolerable to the taste.

Driving Out a Semi-Tertian Fever (*hemitritaeon*)

Semi-Tertian Fever/ Hemitritaeon: A fever that peaks and breaks every day and a half (36 hours, i.e., half of a tertian fever).

 More deadly is the fever which the Greeks call
Hemitritaeon; no one can even say this
In our language, nor did our parents wish us to.
Write many times on a paper the word ABRACADABRA
And repeat it underneath, but take away the final letter
So that more and more single letters are missing from the figure:
You will always take some away, and keep others,
Until a single letter becomes the end of a narrow cone.
Remember: tie this up with a linen thread and bind it to the neck.

---

11   Quintus Serenus, *Liber medicinalis*. This is an original translation by the editor of this volume of the Latin text, which is available at latin.packhum.org.

PART 5

Distilling Classical Medicine in Late Antiquity (ca. 300–700 CE)

Historians in the last several decades, guided especially by Peter Brown of Princeton University (b. 1935), have come to recognize that the traditional date of 476 CE for the "fall" of the Roman Empire does not actually mark a significant divide between "classical" and "medieval" culture. Instead, the later Roman and early Medieval periods in the fourth through eighth centuries are known together as "Late Antiquity," a period in which Christianity became dominant in Europe, Islam was created in the Near East, and both of those religious cultures adopted classical learning. In terms of the history of medicine, Late Antiquity is marked especially by the simplification and codification of the key elements of the Greek and Roman medical traditions.

Diet was always important to ancient medical writers, but it became a central feature of medicine in Late Antiquity and the Middle Ages, partly because of the influence of Galen and his emphasis on food and drink.[1] Since the numbers of professional physicians dwindled significantly in the fourth and fifth centuries CE (particularly in the western Roman Empire), regular foods provided a useful tool for explaining illness and providing cures. Late Antique medical writers recognized the importance of diet to a medical regimen as well as the potentially curative powers of specific foods. This attitude can be seen in the writings of Oribasius (320–403), the personal physician of Emperor Julian the Apostate (r. 361–63) and a prolific author and popularizer of Galen. The passage in Document 34 was copied by Oribasius from a medical text by Antyllus, a Greek doctor from the second century CE. His works are lost apart from excerpts in Oribasius's *Medical Compilations*. Oribasius wrote in Greek but many of his works were translated into Latin during the sixth and seventh centuries, becoming one of the main channels through which medieval European understood basic Galenic medicine before the translations of the High Middle Ages (see Documents 52, pp. 153–57, and 62–66, pp. 188–200).

---

1   See the introduction to Mark Grant, *Galen on Food and Diet* (Routledge, 2000).

Much of Oribasius' dietary information came from Galen and his Roman contemporaries. But after the fall of the Western Roman Empire, the few remaining medical authors tailored their recommendations to a new audience: the Germanic warrior nobility. One such author was Anthimus (Document 35), a Byzantine Greek scholar exiled to the court of Theodoric, Ostrogothic king of Italy, in the sixth century. He wrote a short work in the form of a letter to King Theodoric, recommending or discouraging certain foods. Most of the work is about meat and fish, and there is almost no medical theory explaining why certain foods are good or bad.

The Roman tendency to simplify Greek theoretical medicine continued after the fall of the western empire (476 CE) into the Early Medieval period. Latin bishops like St. Isidore of Seville (ca. 560–636 CE) and Gregory of Tours (see Document 47, pp. 137–38) continued Roman traditions of learning, but primarily for the purpose of providing a basic education for the clergy. Isidore gives a dramatically simplified version of Greco-Roman medical theory in his encyclopedic work *Etymologies* (Document 36), in which all practical applications have been stripped away, leaving only the etymologies of words to form a basic medical education. This work was not intended to teach actual medical practice, but to help a cleric understand the place of medicine and physicians within God's universal order.

The later Roman Empire (ca. 300–500 CE) was a great age for handbooks, which distilled or summarized the learned writings of Greece and Rome at its height. There was a vigorous market for short syntheses of complicated topics, especially medicine. In the fourth century CE a Latin author took the pseudonym *Plinius Secundus Junior* and wrote a brief work called *Medicina Plinii* (*Medicine of Pliny*, Document 37), summarizing the medical passages in Pliny the Elder's first-century work, *Natural History* (Document 32, pp. 98–99). Since the original Pliny did not intend to write a medical treatise, remedies for the same condition are found scattered throughout his encyclopedic work, but the popularity of *Medicine of Pliny* suggests many late Romans found Pliny's medical advice valuable.

While the *Medicine of Pliny* was organized according to ailment to help Romans self-medicate, other works were organized according to plant, like Dioscorides' *De materia medica* (Document 23, pp. 78–79). Just as the author of the *Medicine of Pliny* took a pseudonym, so did the fourth-century author of the *Herbarius* ("herbal"), in Document 38. They claimed to be one Apuleius Platonicus, echoing the fame of both Plato and the second century CE Latin novelist Apuleius of Madaura. Apuleius Platonicus (now commonly called Pseudo-Apuleius) gives his work a mythological foundation, as he claims to have received his knowledge from Chiron the Centaur and Aesculapius (the god Asclepius, see Documents 13–18, pp. 52–61). The herbal describes the effects of 130 different medicinal plants, mostly common natives of

Europe and the Mediterranean, like plantain. Even though Dioscorides was translated into Latin during Late Antiquity, the *Herbarius* was probably the most popular pharmacological work in Europe until it was surpassed by the herbals of Macer Floridus (Document 73, pp. 221–23) and Matthaeus Platearius (Document 75, pp. 226–27) in the twelfth century. It was translated into Old English in the ninth century and later adapted into other vernaculars as well as into Latin poetry in the High Middle Ages (see p. 141 and Document 74, pp. 224–25).

The treatise *De medicamentis* ("On medicines," Document 39) of Marcellus Empiricus is a good example of the continuation and adaptation of older medicine during Late Antiquity. Marcellus lived in Roman Gaul around 400 CE. His nickname *empiricus* reveals his methodology: he claims to have empirically tested or reviewed his medical remedies. In his work he adapted the older herbals by Scribonius Largus and Dioscorides (Document 23, pp. 78–79), adding herbs and cures from his native Gaul. Formal medical education had disappeared by this time in the Western Roman Empire, so Marcellus wrote his book for his compatriots to rely on themselves, testing proposed remedies to see if they actually worked.

Formal medical education still persisted in the Eastern Roman ("Byzantine") Empire after the fall of the West, at least until the Islamic conquests of the seventh century. One of the last representatives of classical Greek medical education was Paul of Aegina, a physician and author active around 640 CE in Alexandria, Egypt, immediately before the Muslim caliph Umar conquered that city in 641. He is known primarily through his voluminous *Seven Books on Medicine*, in which he synthesized ideas from Galen, Oribasius (see Document 34), Aetius of Amida (502–75 CE), and his own medical experience. The passage in Document 40 is typical of theory behind drugs that came to dominate most medieval pharmacology, in both the Latin and Arabic traditions. According to this theory, all medicinal substances (and indeed all food and drink, for that matter) were defined both by their actions within the body, such as cutting, purging, or relaxing the humors. These actions could be identified by taste, and by the relative strength (first through fourth degree or order) of their elemental properties (hot or cold and wet or dry), here called "temperaments."

DOCUMENT 34:
Oribasius: A Galenic Diet in the Later Roman Empire[2]

Oribasius (320–403), the personal physician of Emperor Julian the Apostate (r. 361–63), was a prolific medical author and popularizer of Galen. Most of Oribasius's works are not original, but are carefully designed compilations or paraphrases of older medical works. This passage from Oribasius's *Medical Compilations* comes from a medical text by Antyllus, an otherwise forgotten Greek doctor from the second century CE, who provided detailed dietary recommendations for sick patients.

❧

(1) One must select in the case of continuous illnesses food that is easily digested, quickly distributed around the body, not too nutritious, and excreted without difficulty (for whatever stays in the body revives fevers); bread macerated in water possesses all the above-mentioned qualities. (2) It should be made of three-month wheat, and not too refined (for this sort of food is too nutritious); grind it well and bake it thoroughly. Bread made from the finest quality flour both of this type of wheat and the others should not be eaten because of its strength. Instead the bread should be stale and leavened; soak it in constant changes of hot water, and do not soak all the bread but only the crumb; the part which is like skin in texture is not suitable for successive use and the digestion. A measure of the amount of maceration comes not only from the rising, but also from the breathing of the yeast and the loss of all its smell. (3) Of the same kind are refined groats, and after having had their juice extracted and being sufficiently washed they are boiled and served in water or honeyed milk. (4) Of the same kind too is pearl-barley juice, one part of peeled barley being boiled in fifteen parts of water, a fifth part being left behind after boiling and strained; the juice is drunk while taking at the same time a little honeyed milk. (5) And some people place honeyed milk in a category apart from these foods, although it is boiled down in the same way as we described for pearl-barley, the honey being tempered with a large amount of water equal nearly to a fifth part. (6) The soup from groats is prepared in the following manner: the groats are sufficiently washed, the water in which they are washed being changed often, and once again clean water is poured over them for one hour, and then they are rubbed by hand in the water, until the water is like milk both

---

2 Oribasius, *Medical Compilations* 4.11, in Mark Grant, *Dieting for an Emperor: A Translation of Books 1 and 4 of Oribasius' Medical Compilations with an Introduction and Commentary* (Brill, 1997), 247–51.

in colour and consistency, and then the groats on being filtered in this way remain on the outside; and a little salt to the milky liquid made from the groats, and a small quantity of **dill** in the case of people suffering biting pains in the stomach and inwards, some pennyroyal and thyme for those suffering from an upset stomach and nausea, and some cumin for those suffering from flatulence; boil until there is a degree of solidity and offer before it goes cold. (7) When this sort of food had been well prepared we often prefer [it] to groats and bread because it is easy to administer, is digested without difficulty, and is distributed rapidly in the body. (8) These then are the foods for acute fevers: in difficult circumstances we are often forced through these things not being available or because they are not familiar to the sick people in question, to use other types of food, among which are *itrion*, vegetables, groats, and eggs. *Itrion* should be made from the wheat from which the best baked breads are made; it must be very thin; for when it is thick it bakes unevenly; it must be pounded extremely finely so that it is of the same size as groats; boil in water (especially in rain water, but if not, in the cleanest water possible) for a long time, in order for it to become one single mass through boiling.

dill: Dill is still a common ingredient in gripe water for infants with stomach pains.

DOCUMENT 35:

Anthimus to King Theodoric, *On the Observance of Diet*[3]

After the fall of the Western Roman Empire, the remaining medical authors tailored what they wrote for a new audience: the Germanic warrior nobility. Anthimus was a Byzantine Greek scholar exiled to the court of Theodoric, Ostrogothic king of Italy, in the sixth century. He wrote a short work for Theodoric, recommending or discouraging certain foods, using a dramatically simplified medical theory to justify his choices.

&

Here begins the letter of Anthimus, nobleman, count, and legate for Theodoric, most glorious king of the Franks, concerning the observance of diet.

I have undertaken, so far as I am able, to explain the outline of a diet for Your Piety, that will generally be of benefit for you, according to the teachings of medical authors, since all foods should be eaten so they can be well digested and ensure health, rather than an illness of the stomach or suffering of the human body. The foremost health of men is founded on suitable foods. That is to say, if they were prepared well, they create a good digestion in the body, but if they were not cooked well, they produce heaviness in the stomach and bowels, and even generate heavy humors, and cause slothfulness, painful swellings, and serious belching. From these conditions, vapor rises into the head, whence dizziness and thick fog are apt to occur. Corruption of the bowels will also come from this sort of indigestion, or vomit surely will come up through the mouth, when the stomach should not be able to digest raw foods. But if the foods were well prepared, a good and gentle digestion will result and good humors are nourished. For in this is the best health established, so that those who should wish to manage themselves in such a way will not need other medicines.

Similarly, only as much drink should be taken as agrees with the food. Otherwise, if you eat to excess, and if it is especially cold, the chilled stomach can accomplish nothing. For this reason a corruption arises and those conditions which we named above. Let me provide one example: if someone building the wall of a house mixes lime and water in the proportion demanded for that mixture to thicken, it is beneficial for the fabric of the building and it sets, but if too much water is mixed in, it's no good at all. So also a correct proportion ought to be determined in food and drink.

---

3   *Anthimi de observatione ciborum epistula ad Theudericum regem Francorum*, edited by V. Rose (Teubner, 1877), 7–8, 12–15. Original translation by the editor of this volume.

Therefore, such as we said above, the best health is founded on foods that are cooked well and digested well.

But if someone asks: How can a man on an expedition or taking a long journey manage his diet in such a way? To which I reply, wherever there is a fire or enough time, the aforesaid things can be accomplished. But if necessity demands that you eat meat or other foods raw, don't do it to excess but only sparingly. But what more need I say, since the ancient already said, "**Everything excessive is harmful**." Such is also the case with drink, for if someone going riding or hurrying about on his business should drink too heavily, he will grow sick from the movement on the horse, and even worse things will arise in his bowels than occurred from food.

But perhaps someone will ask me: Why do some other races eat rather raw and bloody meat, and are healthy? It may be that those people are not entirely healthy, because they prepare medicines: when they sense that they are feeling badly, they burn themselves from the fire on the stomach and bowels and other places, just as mad horses are sometimes burned. But I can explain what's happening there. They eat only one food, just like wolves, and not many kinds, because they do not have any food except meat and milk, and they eat whatever they might have. They only seem to be healthy because of this scarcity of food. There is a time when they have something to drink, and a time when they have nothing for a long duration. It is that scarcity which seems to bestow health on them. We, on the other hand, who choke ourselves with a variety of foods and various delights and different drinks, need to govern ourselves in such a way so that we are not aggravated by such excess. Rather, we can obtain health by living more sparingly. But if someone should take delight in eating whatsoever kind of food, let him first take the food prepared well, and then of the other things more sparingly, so he may benefit from what he ate first and digest it well....

Boiled offal of a young cow is a fitting dish. I sometimes allow people to eat the bacon in the stuffing. The liver of a pig, fried, is not at all beneficial for the healthy or the sick, but if the healthy should wish, they should eat it like this: [place it] chopped well on an iron grill which has wide rods, grease it with oil or with fat, and let it roast over the gentle coals until it is rare. Eat it hot, seasoned on top with oil, salt, and coriander....

The flesh of cranes can be eaten sometimes according to desire, because they have dark meat, which produces **black bile**. Plovers are good, especially their breasts, cooked but not roasted. What is more, they are suitable for those who suffer diarrhea or those with dysentery. Therefore let them be boiled well in clean water without any seasoning. And if it is possible, neither salt nor oil should be added, except for one packet of coriander. Cook the [plover breasts] with the [coriander]. Only the breast should be eaten, and without salt if possible. But if that's not possible, just dust it with salt....

Everything excessive is harmful: In Latin, *Omnia nimia nocent*. This phrase was applied as much to medical matters as spiritual, by recommending temperance and moderation in both food and behavior.

black bile: This is a rare example of the application of humoral theory in the Early Middle Ages in Europe.

When salmon is fresh it can be eaten. If it's been around for several days, it injures the stomach. Moreover, if they are salted, they are heavy and nourish bad humors. But if the skin of the salmon has been fried, it should not be eaten at all, because it is seriously harmful. Plaice and sole are of the same kind, and are good and fitting when cooked in salt and oil. They are also fully suitable even for the sick.

DOCUMENT 36:

An Early Medieval Primer in Ancient Medicine by St. Isidore of Seville[4]

St. Isidore (ca. 560–636 CE) was bishop of Seville in Visigothic Spain, where he sought to preserve a simplified form of classical learning in several books, including his encyclopedic *Etymologies*. In the excerpt below from this work, Isidore gives a simplified version of Greco-Roman medical theory, in which the recipes and practical applications have been stripped away, leaving only the etymologies of words to form a basic understanding of medicine.

ex

Medicine. Medicine is that which either aids or restores the health of the body. Its subject matter concerns diseases and wounds. And so there pertain to medicine not only those things displayed by the skill of those, who are properly called physicians, but also food and drink, housing and clothing.

Its Name. Medicine is reckoned to be named from *modus*, "moderation," namely from tempering, so that it is applied not excessively, but little by little. For nature is saddened by too much, but rejoices in moderation. For this reason also those who imbibe **pigmenta** or antidotes too heavily or too often suffer, for all kinds of immoderation produce not health, but danger.

pigmenta: The Latin term for spiced drinks or spices in general. The former is probably meant here.

The Founders of Medicine. The creator or discoverer of the art of medicine is said among the Greeks to be Apollo. His son Aesculapius amplified it through his fame and activities. But after Aesculapius was killed by a lightning bolt, medical skill is said to have been forbidden, and the art passed away along with its creator, and lay hidden for almost 500 years until the time of King Artaxerxes of the Persians. At that time, Hippocrates, son of **Asclepius**, born on the island of Cos, brought medicine back to the light....

Asclepius: It is not clear if this "Asclepius" is simply an alternate spelling of Aesculapius, or if two distinct individuals are meant.

Undertaking the Study of Medicine. Some people ask why the art of medicine is not contained among the other liberal disciplines.[5] The reason is this: they embrace individual subjects, but medicine contains them all. For a doctor ought to know Grammar, so he can understand and explain what he reads. So also Rhetoric, so he can define with truthful arguments the subject he is treating. So also Dialectic, for the purpose of scrutinizing and curing the causes of diseases, through the application of reason. Likewise Arithmetic,

---

4   *Isidori Hispalensis Episcopi Etymologiarum sive Originum libri XX*, edited by W.M. Lindsay, 2 vols. (Oxford: 1911), IV.i–iii, xiii. Original translation by the editor of this volume.

5   Isidore outlines the seven "Liberal Arts," which were first defined by the Roman author Varro (see Document 15, p. 55) and became the basis of formal European education for the next two thousand years. They included the three-part literary *Trivium* of grammar, rhetoric, and dialectic (logic), and the four-part mathematical *Quadrivium* of arithmetic, geometry, music (meaning mathematical musical theory), and astronomy.

on account of the number of hours in the onset of diseases and their daily cycles. It is not otherwise with Geometry, on account of the qualities of regions and the location of places, concerning which he should teach what is fitting for each person to observe. Moreover, Music will not be unknown to him, for there are many things which we read to have happened in sick men through this discipline, such as is read about David, who snatched Saul away from the unclean spirit by the art of musical modulation. Asclepiades the healer also restored a certain person in a frenzy to his original health using a *symphonia*. Finally, he will have an understanding of Astronomy, through which he may contemplate the order of the stars and the changing of the seasons. For, as a certain physician said, our bodies are changed together with the **qualities of the seasons**. For these reasons Medicine is called a second Philosophy, for each discipline claims all of man for itself. For just as the soul is cured by Philosophy, so the body is cured through Medicine.

symphonia: The source of the modern English word "symphony," but it referred to various individual instruments in classical and medieval Latin.

qualities of the seasons: An allusion to the Hippocratic work *Airs, Waters, Places* (Document 11, pp. 42–45).

DOCUMENT 37:
Medicine of Pliny for the Informed Traveler[6]

In the fourth century a Latin author under the pseudonym of *Plinius Secundus Junior* ("younger follower of Pliny") wrote a brief work, *Medicine of Pliny*, to summarize the medical passages in Pliny the Elder's first-century work, *Natural History* (Document 32, pp. 98–99). *Plinius Secundus Junior* organized the recipes found in *Natural History* according to the ailment treated. He claims to have done this for the use of travelers lest they be deceived by unscrupulous healers.

e

Prologue. It frequently happens that while I'm travelling I experience the various frauds of healers, either on account of my own illness or those of my companions. They sell the most vile remedies for huge prices, and some of them undertake those cases which they don't know how to cure, for the sake of greed. In fact, I have heard that some of them act in such a fashion that they even prolong ailments, which could be removed in a very few days or even hours, for a long time, so they hold on to their patients just for the money. They make themselves more dangerous than the diseases they treat. Therefore it seemed necessary to me that I gather together from all parts aids for health and collect them in a sort of notebook, so that wherever I should go, I could avoid snares of this sort and pursue my travels from this time on with this assurance, that I know, if some ailment should befall me, that they won't make any money off of me nor will they even find an opportunity....

For a Headache. A headache is relieved if you thoroughly mix two spoonfuls of the juice of a cut leek and one of honey and pour this either into the nostrils or into the ears. Chronic pain and vertigo are cured by the juice of the black beet, rubbed on the temples. A very useful cure for pain is when the head is smeared with the juice of *intibus* with rose oil and vinegar; basil in rose oil, myrtle oil, or vinegar if applied to the forehead; rue is drunk with wine; and the juice of ground rue is dripped into the head with vinegar or rose oil. Applying the crown of the pennyroyal plant is beneficial. It is suitable for the forehead to be sprinkled and rubbed with a mixture of egg white, wheat flour, and a little white salt, and wrapped with a foot-long bandage. Dill is plucked from the garden to be used like this: it is cooked in oil and an ache is rubbed with its juice. Creeping thyme, cooked in vinegar, is rubbed

intibus: This name, or *intubus*, was used for several edible, leafy greens such as chicory and endive.

---

6 *Plinii Secundi Iunioris qui feruntur de medicina libri tres*, edited by Alf Önnerfors, Corpus medicorum latinorum 3 (Berlin, 1964), 4–5, 7–8. Original translation by the editor of this volume.

on the forehead and temples. And if it is difficult to sleep, it is good to rub the head all over with almond oil. Rub painful temples with boiled garlic.

DOCUMENT 38:
The *Herbarius* of Apuleius Platonicus[7]

The fourth-century author of this *Herbarius* (herbal) took the pseudonym Apuleius Platonicus, echoing the fame of both Plato and the second-century CE Latin author Apuleius of Madaura (125–170 CE). Apuleius Platonicus (or Pseudo-Apuleius) describes the effects of 130 different medicinal plants. To help his readers identify this plant in other books, or perhaps in marketplaces, Pseudo-Apuleius provides numerous synonyms for each herb. Thanks to the continuing popularity of the *Herbarius*, these alternate plant names passed down into medieval herbalism long after they were still used to identify the plants.

The Herbal of Apuleius Platonicus, which he received from Chiron the Centaur, teacher of Achilles, and from Aesculapius.

Apuleius Platonicus to his fellow citizens:

Out of many public monuments, I have delivered up to the witness of truth just a few of the powers of herbs and the cures for bodies, because of the wordy senselessness of the medical profession. We call this the boasting of doctors rather than their cures, and in truth we often call those men the children of ineptitude and lack of learning, money-grubbers to be sure, who seek payment even from the dead. What do they do? Nothing. For they wait for an occasion and go back and forth, and while they draw out the time of medical treatment, they become, I reckon, more dangerous than the diseases themselves. Therefore let us display the titles of the dead, that time assemble them together, now especially, so that our literary knowledge may seem to benefit those of my fellow citizens, whether indeed companions or travelers, whom any bodily trouble has afflicted, even if the doctors are unwilling.

The Herb Plantain

1. For headache. The root of the herb plantain, hung from the neck, marvelously removes a headache.

---

7   E. Howald and H.E. Sigerist, *Antonii Musae de herba vettonica liber. Pseudoapulei herbarius. Anonymi de taxone liber. Sexti Placiti liber medicinae ex animalibus....* Corpus medicorum latinorum, 4 (Leipzig-Berlin, 1927), 15, 22–25. Original translation by the editor of this volume.

2. For stomachache. The juice of plantain, when warmed and applied as a compress, takes away a stomachache, and if there should be swellings, when it is ground and applied, it takes away the swelling.

3. For internal pains. The juice of plantain, given in a drink, heals interior matters and marvelously purges a person's torso.

4. For those with dysentery. Cook plantain with lentils and give it [to the patient], let him eat: it restrains the belly.

5. Those who excrete foul matter with blood. Order them to drink the juice of plantain, and they will be healed.

6. For wounds. The ground seed of plantain, sprinkled in a wound, quickly heals wounds, and when it is ground and applied cools those places, which were burning with excessive heat, and thoroughly heals them.

7. For restraining the bowels. Cook plantain with vinegar and let it be drunk with unmixed wine at the measure of one glass.

8. For snakebite. The herb plantain, ground and taken with wine, will be suitable.

9. For scorpion bite. It is believed that the root of plantain, when bound [to the bite], is marvelously beneficial.

10. For worms. Grind up plantain and give one spoonful or *ligula* of its juice to drink, and also apply the ground herb around the navel.

11. If there should be any hardening in the body. Cook plantain in grease without salt and make it into a poultice: apply it to the hardening and this breaks it up.

12. For quartan fevers. When the juice of the herb plantain, in honey water, is given two hours before the attack [of the fever], you will marvel at the outcome.

13. For gout and any pain or swelling of the nerves. The leaves of plantain, bruised or baked with a little salt and applied, is certain to work very well.

14. For tertian fevers. Grind up three roots of plantain, give it to the fasting [patient] before the attack [of the fever] with wine or water, and have him drink.

15. For the pain of afterbirth. The seed of plantain, ground and given in a drink, is considered beneficial.

16. For recent wounds. Plantain, ground and applied with old grease without salt, is rendered curative.

17. If your feet are swollen from travel. Plantain, ground and applied with vinegar, relieves the swelling.

18. If an ulcer should arise below the eye or the nose. The expressed juice of ground plantain is rendered curative when one applies soft wool infused with the juice for nine days.

19. For the dysenteric or colicky. Give plantain seed, ground with barley flour, in hot wine, let him drink and he will be made healthy.
20. For abscesses. Plantain with old grease, baked and applied, heals completely.
21. For mouth sores. The juice and leaves of plantain are held in the mouth and its roots are chewed in the mouth.
22. For healing fistulas. The juice of plantain is poured or inserted into the fistulas.
23. For the bite of a rabid dog. Plantain, when bruised and applied, heals most readily.
24. Against all difficulties urinating. When the leaves or roots of plantain are drunk with raisin wine, it is highly curative.

Names of the herb. It is called *arnoglossa* by the Greeks, others call it *arnion*, others *probation*, others *cinoglossa*, others *eptapleuron*, the Gauls call it *tarbidolotius*, the Spanish *tetharica*, Sicilians *polineuron*, others *torsion*, the prophets call it *ura egneumonos*, the Egyptians *asaer*, others *thetarion*, Dacians *sipoax*, Italians call it broad plantain, Romans call it greater plantain, others *septeneruia*. It grows most often in marshy places and fields.

DOCUMENT 39:
Marcellus and His Empirical Handbook of Medicines[8]

Marcellus lived in Roman Gaul around 400 CE, where he wrote the treatise *De medicamentis* (*On medicines*). He was given the nickname *Empiricus* because he claims to have empirically tested or reviewed his medical remedies. The passage below is the prologue to his book, in which he lays out the reasons why and methods by which he compiled a new medical handbook.

❧

Marcellus, Nobleman, Ex-Magister of the Offices of Theodosius the Old, sends greetings to his son: Imitating the example of those zealous men, who, although strangers to the rules of medicine, have nevertheless exercised noble care for causes of this sort, I have written this book concerning empirical medicines, with as much care and diligence as I can muster, containing the preparation of remedies, founded in natural philosophy or reason, and notes about them from here and there. For if I have ever obtained knowledge of anything suitable for health and for the curing of people, either from others, or I myself have tested it by use, or understood it by reading, I have gathered it, at first scattered and detached, and reassembled it into one body—just like Aesculapius gathering the scattered and mangled limbs of **Virbius**.

I have dug up, through my reading, not only the ancient authors on the art of medicine writing, to be sure, in the Latin language, such as the works of either **Pliny, Apuleius, Celsus, Apollinaris**, and **Designatianus**, and some other men from a nearer time, famous for their honors, fellow citizens and our elders, Siburius, Eutropius, and Ausonius, but I have also learned some remedies, simple ones and by chance, from farmers and peasants, which I have tested by experience. I have undertaken a most pious vow, dearest sons, to supply an abundance of their writings to you, through our labor long nights, for the sake of human infirmity; and I pray above all to divine mercy that no need arise for you or your loved ones ever to need this book, but if any cause should occur for you to search for healing and to strengthen your health, I pray that this will provide for you the necessary aid and cure, without the intercession of a doctor. And you ought to communicate the benefits of this knowledge, by a mutual exchange of human love, for the care of all sickly friends, known or unknown, but above all to

Virbius: A Roman forest god, identified with the Greek figure Hippolytus, son of Theseus.

Pliny, Apuleius, Celsus: See Documents 28 (pp. 91–92), 38 (pp. 113–15) and 25 (pp. 83–85) respectively for more on these Latin medical authors.

Apollinaris: Possibly Marcellus' fellow Gallo-Roman, Sidonius Apollinaris, a renowned Latin poet and bishop, although he is not known for any medical writings.

Designatianus: Largius Designatianus, a fourth-century CE Latin medical writer who is now known only through Marcellus' work.

---

8   Marcellus Empiricus, *Marcelli de medicamentis liber*, edited by M. Niedermann and E. Liechtenhan, German translation by J. Kollesch and D. Nickel, 2 vols., Corpus medicorum latinorum V (Berlin, 1968), 2–4. Original translation by the editor of this volume.

strangers and to the poor, because the mercy which is shown to a sick guest or a needy pilgrim is more agreeable to God and more praiseworthy to men. To be sure, I warn you, that if any medicines must be prepared, you do not prepare them carelessly without a doctor, or keep them without diligence.

For although I have most attentively chosen the nature of the drugs and their dose for each remedy; and although I have placed at the head of this book the signs of the measures and the value of the weights according to the tradition of the Greeks and the practice of the ancient physicians; and I have given this explanation not only in Roman, but also in Greek explanation, nevertheless it is important that these measures are verified by more skillful people and often corrected, and that the remedies, once compounded or prepared, are always preserved under seals, because an accident could occur or someone's malevolence disturb them. That which was prepared sincerely and with good intention may corrupt, a poison may be made from a remedy, disaster may come from healthfulness, and medicine may be blamed, when lack of prudence has erred.

In conclusion, let it suffice that I have prepared these recipes for you in a kindly fashion, but that I also have warned you about these matters; and let it be equally fitting that you deliberate on both your own health and my advice. I added to this work, so that it was complete, the letters of those whose zeal served as an example: the reading of these may urge you on to a necessary understanding and instruct you in the ways of health....[9]

9   As Marcellus promised, he begins his work with a description of measurements and weights found in the works of Hippocrates and Pliny the Elder, followed by a series of genuine and spurious classical letters on medical themes, such as letters from Hippocrates to King Antiochus and his friend Maecenas. Marcellus also reproduces the prologue to the *Medicine of Pliny* (Document 37, pp. 111–12), which he believed to have been written by the real Pliny the Elder (Document 32, pp. 98–99).

DOCUMENT 40:
The Drug Theory of Paul of Aegina[10]

Paul of Aegina was a physician and author active around 640 CE in Alexandria, Egypt. In his *Seven Books on Medicine* he synthesized ideas from Galen, Oribasius (see Document 34, pp. 104–05), Aetius of Amida (502–75 CE), and his own medical experience. In this passage Paul outlines the theory of "temperaments" (elemental qualities of hot or cold and wet and dry) by which he defined medicines and gauged their strength. Variations on this pharmacological system were used for the rest of the Middle Ages in Latin Europe and Islamicate lands.

e

On the Temperaments of Substances as Indicated by Their Tastes

It is not safe to judge from the smell with regard to the temperament of sensible objects; for inodorous substances consist indeed of thick particles, but it is not clear whether they are of a hot or cold nature; and odorous substances, to a certain extent, consist of fine particles and are hot; but the degree of the smallness of their parts, or of their hotness, is not indicated, because of the inequality of their substance. And still more impracticable is it to judge of them from their colors, for of every color are found hot, cold, drying, and moistening substances. But in tasting, all parts of the bodies subjected to it come in contact with the tongue and excite the sense, so that thereby one may judge clearly of their powers in their temperaments. Astringents, then, contract, obstruct, condense, dispel, and thicken; and, in addition to all these properties, they are of a cold and drying nature. That which is acid, cuts, divides, thins, removes obstructions, and cleanses without heating; but that which is acrid, resembles the acid in being thinning and purgative, but differs from it in this, that the acid is cold, and the acrid is hot; and, further, in this, that the acid repels, but the acrid attracts, consumes, breaks down, and helps form scabs. In like manner, that which is bitter cleanses the pores, is cleansing and thinning, and cuts the thick humors without a perceptible heat. What is watery is cold, thick, condenses, contracts, obstructs, deadens, and dulls. But that which is salty contracts, braces, preserves as a pickle, and dries without noticeable heat or cold. What is sweet relaxes, **concocts**, softens, and rarefies; but what is oily moistens, softens, and relaxes.

concocts: Coction or concoction is the "cooking" of humors within the body, sometimes beneficial (as with the growth of children) and sometimes harmful (as with the corruption of humors leading to dangerous diseases).

---

10 Adapted from *The Seven Books of Paulus Ægineta*, translation and commentary by Francis Adams, 3 vols. (The Sydenham Society, 1844), Vol. 3, 1–2.

On the Order and Degrees of the Temperaments

A moderate medicine which is of the same temperament as that to which it is applied, so as neither to dry, moisten, cool, nor heat, must not be called either dry, moist, cold, or hot; but whatever is drier, moister, hotter, or colder, is so called from its prevailing power. It will be sufficient for every useful purpose to make four degrees according to the prevailing temperament, calling the substance hot, according to the first degree, when it heats, indeed, but not perceptibly, requiring reflection to demonstrate its existence: and in like manner with regard to cold, dry, and moist, when the prevailing temperament requires demonstration, and has no strong nor manifest virtue. Such things as are manifestly possessed of drying, moistening, heating or cooling properties, may be said to be of the second degree. Such things as have these properties to a strong, but not an extreme degree, may be said to be of the third degree. But such things as are naturally so hot as to form scars or to burn, are of the fourth. In like manner such things as are so cold as to occasion the death of a body part are also of the fourth degree. But nothing is of so drying a nature as to be of the fourth degree, without burning, for that which dries in a great degree burns also; such are chalcopyrite, rock alum, and quicklime. But a substance may be of the third rank of desiccants without being caustic, such as all those things which are strongly astringent, of which kind are the unripe juice of grapes, sumac, and alum.

PART 6

Medical Diversity in the Early Middle Ages (ca. 600–1000 CE)

MONOTHEISM AND MEDICINE (DOCUMENTS 41–45)

C lassical Greece and Rome were essentially polytheistic societies, their people worshipping a large number of gods and gladly embracing new ones from neighboring cultures (in a combination of tolerance and imperialism). The monotheistic Jews were only a small minority in the Roman Empire, but their religion would come to inspire the two other great monotheistic religions, Christianity and Islam, whose followers now make up roughly half of the world's population. Christianity was legalized in 311 CE by the Roman Emperors Constantine and Galerius. By the end of the fourth century, it was the official religion of the Empire and received significant financial and political support. Islam arose during the early seventh century CE, through the preaching and conquests of Muhammad and his followers. Therefore, by about 700 CE, almost the entire former Greco-Roman world was monotheist in one form or another. Jews, Christians, and Muslims all adopted ancient Greek medicine but sought ways to adapt it to their monotheistic religions. Usually this wasn't difficult, but sometimes the writings of Hippocrates, Galen, and other ancient pagan physicians included elements that were offensive to belief in one, all-powerful God. For example, both medieval Jews and Christians prepared medical oaths to replace or modify the pagan elements of the Hippocratic *Oath*. The Jewish physicians Asaph and Yohanan wrote the explicitly monotheistic *Oath of Asaph* sometime between the fourth and sixth centuries CE in the Eastern Roman Empire. Likewise, Greek Christians modified the Hippocratic *Oath* at some point in the Early Middle Ages, replacing the Greek gods with the Christian God and Christ. In an image from a twelfth-century Greek manuscript (Document 42), the Christian aspect of this revised oath is emphasized further by writing it in the shape of a cross.

One of the key Christian institutions to develop in the Early Middle Ages was monasticism, the establishment of religious communities of monks or nuns, who lived their entire lives in prayer and holy labor, often according to a strict rule. Numerous monastic rules were written during the fourth through sixth centuries, but the most influential by far was the *Rule of St. Benedict* (Document 43), which Benedict of Nursia prepared around 535 CE for a group of monks in Italy. Benedict's rule was eventually adopted throughout medieval Europe and is used to this day in Christian monastic communities around the world. Benedict's rule appealed to many communities because it was satisfyingly strict while remaining more humane and manageable than some of the most rigorous rules. Because some monks were expected to spend their entire lives in a monastery, Benedict dedicated several chapters to their medical care and moderate diet.

Almost all Christian saints were believed to have the ability to heal, a miraculous power granted to them by God before or after death. This healing power is often explicitly non-medical and succeeds where secular medicine and doctors have failed. Only a few saints, therefore, were said to be engaged in secular medical care as physicians. Two of the most famous are the brothers Cosmas and Damian, early Syrian or Arab Christians who were martyred for their faith during the reign of Emperor Diocletian (r. 284–305 CE). Cosmas and Damian were famous in life for their medical skill. They and their three other brothers were called before the proconsul, a Roman official, and ordered to make sacrifices to pagan idols. As Christians, they refused, and were consequently tortured and crucified. They performed miracles after their deaths, in answer to the prayers of the sick, and appeared in dreams much like Asclepius (see Documents 13–18, pp. 52–61). Churches dedicated to Saints Cosmas and Damian were founded as early as the fourth century and their story was told throughout the Middle Ages. The version in Document 44 comes from the *Legenda Aurea* (*Golden Legend*), one of the most popular collections of saints' lives from the Middle Ages. Compiled by the Dominican friar Jacobus de Voragine around the year 1260, *The Golden Legend* contains several hundred stories of Christian saints from the earliest days of the faith up to Jacobus's own time.

The Jewish and Christian Bibles were composed over centuries and contain separate books in a variety of genres. The Islamic Quran, on the other hand, was most likely composed far more quickly from the revelations of Muhammad in the period 610–32 CE, and written down soon after that. Muslims look to the Prophet Muhammad and their holiest book for guidance in all matters of life, including medicine, but there is little specifically about disease or healing in the Quran. An important exception is Quran 26:80, "There is no disease that God Almighty has created, except that He also has created its treatment." This verse was widely accepted as divine approval for human medicine and the investigation of disease. After the Quran, the most revered religious texts for Muslims are the *hadith*, records of the saying and actions of the Prophet Muhammad and his companions.

Soon after the death of Muhammad in 632 CE, his followers began to gather these *hadith*, which were eventually codified in collections known as *sunan* (plural of *sunnah*, "tradition"). The *Sunan Abu Dawud* (Document 45), for example, was compiled during the ninth century by the Persian Muslim jurist Abu Dawud. One of the books in this collection, the *Kitab al-Tibb*, is dedicated to the Prophet's sayings about medicine.

DOCUMENT 41:

The Oath of Asaph, a Jewish Physician's Oath[1]

The Hebrew *Oath of Asaph* is similar in form and content to the ancient
Greek Hippocratic *Oath* (Document 13, pp. 52–53), but it was written by and
for Jews. It is ascribed to two Jewish physicians named Asaph and Yohanan,
who lived sometime in the fourth to sixth centuries CE, probably in Israel
under the rule of the Eastern Roman (Byzantine) Empire. The *Oath of Asaph*
is found in several copies of a medical compilation known as the *Sefer 'Asaph*,
"Book of Asaph," the oldest medical book in Hebrew and one of the few
available in that language before the High Middle Ages (see Document 84,
pp. 247–48).

ꝛ

This is the pact which Asaph ben Berakhyahu and Yohanan ben Zabda
made with their pupils, and they adjured them with the following words:
Do not attempt to kill any soul by means of a potion of herbs, Do not make
a woman [who is] pregnant [as a result] of whoring take a drink with a view
to causing **abortion**, Do not covet beauty of form in women with a view to
fornicating with them, Do not divulge the secret of a man who has trusted
you, Do not take any reward [which may be offered in order to induce you]
to destroy and to ruin, Do not harden your heart [and turn it away] from
pitying the poor and healing the needy, Do not say of [what is] good; it is
bad, nor of [what is] bad: it is good, Do not adopt the ways of the sorcerers
using [as they do] charms, augury and sorcery in order to separate a man
from the wife of his bosom or a woman from the companion of her youth,
You shall not covet any wealth or reward [which may be offered in order to
induce you] to help in a lustful desire, You shall not seek help in any idola-
trous [worship] so as to heal through [a recourse to idols], and you shall not
heal with anything [pertaining] to their worship, But on the contrary detest
and abhor and hate all those who worship them, put their trust in them,
and give assurance [referring] to them, For they are all naught, useless, for
they are nothing, demons, spirits of the dead; they cannot help their own
corpses, how then could they help those who live?

Now [then] put your trust in the Lord, your God, [who is] a true God, a
living God, For [it is] He who kills and makes alive, who wounds and heals,
Who teaches men knowledge and also to profit, Who wounds with justice

> **abortion:** As with the
> Hippocratic *Oath*, the
> meaning here is the
> intentional abortion of an
> unwanted fetus, rather than
> an accidental miscarriage,
> which can be the meaning
> of "abortion" in many
> premodern texts.

---

1   Shlomo Pines, "The Oath of Asaph the Physician and Yohanan ben Zabda, Its Relation to the
    Hippocratic Oath and the *Doctrina duarum viarum* of the Didache," *Proceedings of the Israel
    Academy of Science and Humanities* 5 (1971–76), 223–64: 224–26.

and righteousness, and who heals with pity and compassion, No designs of [His] sagacity are beyond His [power], And nothing is hidden from His eyes.

Who causes curative plants to grow, Who puts sagacity into the hearts of the wise in order that they should heal through the abundance of His loving-kindness, and that they should recount wonders in the congregation of many; so that every living [being] knows that He made him and that there is no saviour [other] than He. For the nations trust in their idols, who [are supposed] to save them from their distress and will not deliver them from their misfortunes, For their trust and hope is in the dead. For this [reason] it is fitting to keep yourselves separate from them; to remove yourselves and keep far away from all the abominations of their idols, And to cleave to the name of the Lord God of spirits for all flesh, And the soul of every living being is in His hand to kill and to make live, And there is none that can deliver out of His hand.

Remember Him always and seek Him in truth, in righteousness in an upright way, in order that you should prosper in all your works, And He will give you help to make you prosper in [what you are doing], and you shall be [said to be] happy in the mouth of all flesh. And the nations will abandon their idols and images and will desire to worship God like you, For they will know that their trust is in vain and their endeavor fruitless, For they implore a god, who will not do good [to them], who will not save [them].

As for you, be strong, do not let your hands be weak, for your work shall be rewarded, The Lord is with you, while you are with Him, If you keep His pact, follow His commandments, cleaving to them, You will be regarded as His saints in the eyes of all flesh, and they will say: Happy the people whose [lot] is such, happy the people whose God is the Lord.

Their pupils answered saying: We will do all that you exhorted and ordered us [to do], For it is a commandment of the Torah, And we must do it with all our heart, with all our soul and with all our might, To do and to obey, Not to swerve or turn aside to the right hand or the left, And they [Asaph and Yohanan] blessed them in the name of God most high, maker of heaven and earth.

And they continued to charge them, and said: The Lord God, His saints and His Torah [bear] witness, that you should fear Him, that you should not turn aside from His commandments, and that you should follow His laws with an upright heart, You shall not incline after lucre [so as] to help a godless [man in shedding] innocent blood. You shall not mix a deadly drug for any man or woman so that he [or she] should kill their fellow-man. You shall not speak of the herbs [out of which such drugs are made]. You shall not hand them over to any man, And you shall not talk about any matter [connected] with this, You shall not use blood in any work of medicine, You shall not attempt to provoke an ailment in a human soul through [the use of] iron instruments or searing with fire before making an examination two or three times; then [only] should you give your advice. You shall not be ruled—your eyes and your heart being lifted up—by a haughty spirit. Do not keep [in your hearts] the vindictiveness of hatred with regard to a sick man, You shall not change your words in anything, The Lord our God hates [this] being done, But keep His orders and commandments, and follow all His ways, in order to please Him, [and] to be pure, true and upright.

Thus did Asaph and Yohanan exhort and adjure their pupils.

DOCUMENT 42:

A Christianized Hippocratic *Oath* (Greek, twelfth century CE)[2]

Throughout the medieval period, Latin and Greek Christians, Jews, and Muslims all embraced the teachings of Hippocrates. However, the Hippocratic *Oath* (Document 13, pp. 52–53) was unacceptable in its original form as it called on pagan gods for witness and support. At some point in the Early Middle Ages, Greek scholars changed the wording of the oath and replaced the gods Apollo, Asclepius, Hygieia, and Panacea with Christ alone.[3] In the image below, made during the twelfth century in a Greek-speaking area of Italy, the Christianized oath has even been written in the shape of a cross and given a new title: "From the Oath According to Hippocrates in so far as a Christian May Swear It."[4]

---

2   Vatican City, Bibliotheca Apostolica Vaticana, MS Urb. Gr. 64, fol. 116r, early 12th c., Calabria or Sicily.

3   Vivian Nutton, *Ancient Medicine*, 2nd ed. (Routledge, 2013), 415 n87.

4   W.H.S. Jones, *The Doctor's Oath: An Essay in the History of Medicine* (Cambridge UP, 1924), 23, 25.

DOCUMENT 43:

Medicine and Diet in the *Rule of St. Benedict*[5]

Mediterranean Christians first established monasteries and monastic rules in the fourth and fifth centuries CE, so that a special few men and women could lead lives of prayer and holy labor. The most influential monastic rule was written by St. Benedict of Nursia around 535 CE in Italy. Benedict dedicated several chapters of the *Rule* to the medical care and moderate diet of the monks, who cared for their sick brothers and for sick pilgrims in imitation of Christ himself.

ev

Chapter XXXVI: Of the Sick Brethren

Before all things, and above all things, special care must be taken of the sick, so that they be served in very deed, as Christ Himself, for He saith: "I was sick, and ye visited Me." And: "What ye did to one of these My least Brethren, ye did to Me." But let the sick themselves bear in mind that they are served for the honour of God, and must not grieve the Brethren who serve them by their extravagant demands. Nevertheless, they must patiently be borne with, because there is gotten from such a more abundant reward. Therefore let the Abbot take special care they be not neglected.

Let a separate cell be set apart for their use, and an attendant that is God-fearing, diligent, and careful. As often as it shall be expedient, let the use of baths be allowed the sick; but to such as are in health, and especially to the young, let it be seldom granted. Moreover the sick and weakly may be allowed the use of flesh meat for their recovery. As soon, however, as they get better, they must all, after the accustomed manner, abstain from meat. Let the Abbot take special care that the Cellarer or attendants neglect not the sick, because whatever is done amiss by his disciplines, is imputed to himself.

Chapter XXXIX: Of the Measure or Quantity of Meat

We think it sufficient for daily refection, both at the sixth and ninth hour, that there be at all seasons two dishes, because of the infirmities of different people; so that he who cannot eat of one, may make his meal of the other. Let therefore two dishes of hot food suffice for the Brethren, and if there be any apples or young vegetables, let them be added as a third dish. Let one pound weight of bread suffice for the day, whether there be one refection,

---

5   *The Rule of Our Most Holy Father St. Benedict, Patriarch of Monks* (London, 1875), 159, 161, 169, 171.

or both dinner and supper. If they are to sup, let a third part of that pound be reserved by the Cellarer, to be put before them at supper.

If their labour be great, it shall be in the power of the Abbot to add what he shall think fitting to their ordinary allowance; taking care always to avoid excess and surfeiting, that the Monks be not overtaken with indigestion, because there is no sin more contrary to a Christian than gluttony, as our Lord saith: "Take heed to yourselves lest perhaps your hearts be overcharged with surfeiting and drunkenness." But to children of tender age, let not the same quantity be given, but less than to the older, in all things preserving moderation and frugality. Let all, except the very weak and the sick, abstain from eating the flesh of four footed beasts.

DOCUMENT 44:

Roman Doctors as Christian Saints: Cosmas and Damian[6]

Hagiography, or the writing of saints' lives, is one of the most valuable sources for understanding medieval Christianity. Thousands of medieval saints' lives survive and many of those saints performed miraculous healing. Saints Cosmas and Damian, however, are rare among saints for also being practicing physicians who cured using both natural and miraculous means. According to their *vita* (saint's life), Cosmas and Damian were martyred for their faith during the persecutions of Emperor Diocletian (r. 284–305 CE). Churches dedicated to Saints Cosmas and Damian appear as early as the fourth century and their story was told throughout the Middle Ages. The version below is late, coming from the *Legenda Aurea* (*The Golden Legend*), a collection of saints' lives compiled by the Dominican friar Jacobus de Voragine around the year 1260 as a resource for preachers.

e

Cosmas and Damian were brethren germane, that is of one father and of one mother, and were of the city Egea, and born of a religious mother named Theodora. They were learned in the art of medicine, and of leechcraft, and received so great grace of God that they healed all maladies and languors, not only of men but also cured and healed beasts. And did all for the love of God without taking of any reward. There was a lady which had spent all her goods in medicines, and came to these saints, and anon was healed of her sickness, and then she offered a little gift to St. Damian, but he would not receive it. And she swore and conjured him by horrible oaths that he granted to receive it, and not for covetousness of the gift, but for to obey to the devotion of her that offered it, and that he would not be seen to despise the name of our Lord of which he had been conjured. And when St. Cosmas knew it, he commanded that his body should not be laid after his death with his brother's. And the night following our Lord appeared to St. Cosmas and excused his brother. And when Lysias heard their renown he made them to be called to him, and demanded their names and their country. And then the holy martyrs said: Our names be Cosmas and Damian, and we have three other brethren which be named Antimas, Leontius, and Euprepius, our country is Arabia, but Christian men know not fortune. Then the proconsul or judge commanded them that they should bring forth their brethren, and

---

6   Jacobus de Voragine, *The Golden Legend: Or, Lives of the Saints*, translated by William Caxton, 7 vols. (London, 1900), Vol. 5, 172–77. Modified.

that they should all together do sacrifice to the idols.... And they suffered death under Diocletian about the year of our Lord 287.

... It happened that a husbandman after he had labored in the field about reaping of his corn, he slept with open mouth in the field, and a serpent entered by his mouth into his body. Then he awoke and felt nothing, and after returned into his house. And at evening he began to be tormented and cried piteously, and called unto his help the holy saints of God, Cosmas and Damian, and when the pain and anguish increased he went to the church of the saints, and then the serpent issued out of his mouth like it had entered.

... Felix, the eighth pope after St. Gregory, did do make a noble church at Rome of the saints Cosmas and Damian, and there was a man who served devoutly the holy martyrs in that church, who a cancer had consumed all his thigh. And as he slept, the holy martyrs Cosmas and Damian, appeared to him their devout servant, bringing with them an instrument and ointment of whom that one said to that other: "Where shall we have flesh when we have cut away the rotten flesh to fill the voice place?" Then that other said to him: "There is an Ethiopian that this day is buried in the churchyard of St. Peter ad Vincula, which is yet fresh, let us bear this thither, and take we out of the **Moor**'s flesh and fill this place with it. And so they fetched the thigh of the sick man and so changed that one for the other. And when the sick man awoke and felt no pain, he put forth his hand and felt his leg without hurt, and then took a candle, and saw well that it was not his thigh, but that it was another. And when he was well come to himself, he sprang out of his bed for joy, and recounted to all the people how it happened to him, and that which he had seen in his sleep, and how he was healed. And they sent hastily to the tomb of the dead man, and found the thigh of him cut off, and that other thigh in his tomb instead of his.

Then let us pray unto these holy martyrs to be our succour and help in all our hurts, wounds and sores, and that by their merits after this life we may come to everlasting bliss in heaven. Amen.

Moor: An ancient and medieval European term for North Africans, especially the Berbers. In later centuries it was used to refer to any African Muslims.

DOCUMENT 45:

Islamic Medicine of the Prophet: *Sunan Abu Dawud*[7]

The *Sunan Abu Dawud* (also *Dawood*) is one of the earliest and most important collections of Islamic *hadith*, or statements attributed to Muhammad and his early companions, gathered as supplements to the religious authority of the Quran. It was compiled during the ninth century by the Persian Muslim jurist Abu Dawud (d. 889 CE), who collected about 5,000 *hadith* into 36 categories. One book, the *Kitab al-Tibb*, is dedicated to the Prophet's sayings about medicine, which attribute to Muhammad dietary and medical knowledge.

e

Book 22: The Book of Medicine

Chapter 1459: A Man Should Seek a Remedy

Usamah b. Sharik said: I came to the Prophet (may peace be upon him) and his Companions were sitting as if they had birds on their heads. I saluted and sat down. The desert Arabs then came from here and there. They asked: Apostle of Allah, should we make use of medical treatment? He replied: Make use of medical treatment, for Allah has not made a disease without appointing a remedy for it, with the exception of one disease, namely old age....

Chapter 1460: Prevention

Umm al-Mundhar, daughter of Qais al-Ansariyyah said: The Apostle of Allah (may peace be upon him) came to visit me accompanied by 'Ali who was convalescing. We had some ripe dates hung up. The Apostle of Allah (may peace be upon him) got up and began to eat from them. 'Ali also got up to eat, but the Apostle of Allah (may peace be upon him) kept on saying to 'Ali: Stop, 'Ali, for you are convalescing, and 'Ali stopped. She said: I then prepared some barley and beet-root and brought it. The Apostle of Allah (may peace be upon him) then said: Take some of this, 'Ali, for it will be more beneficial for you.

---

7   Adapted from *English Translation of Sunan Abu Dawud*, translated by Nasiruddin al-Khattab, reviewed by Abû Khaliyi, 5 vols. (Darussalam, 2008), Vol. 4, 305–09.

Chapter 1461: Cupping

Abu Hurairah reported the Apostle of Allah (may peace be upon him) as saying: The best medical treatment you apply is **cupping**.

Salmah, the maid-servant of the Apostel of Allah (may peace be upon him), said: No one complained to the Apostle of Allah (may peace be upon him) of a headache but he told him to get himself cupped, or of a pain in his legs but he told him to **dye them with henna**.

Chapter 1463: Dates on Which it is Commendable to Get Oneself Cupped

... Jabir said: The Apostle of Allah (may peace be upon him) had himself cupped above the thigh for a contusion from which he suffered.

Chapter 1464: Cutting of a Vein and Place of Cupping

Jabir said: The Prophet (may peace be upon him) sent a physician to Ubayy (b. Ka'b), and he cut his vein.

cupping: The application of heated glasses to specific points on a patient's skin for the purpose of drawing out or shifting the internal humors.

dye them with henna: Apply henna or a similar skin dye as a medical treatment.

EARLY MEDIEVAL RESPONSES TO PLAGUE AND PESTILENCE (DOCUMENTS 46–48)

The belief that plagues were spread through polluted air was one of the most common natural explanations during antiquity and the Middle Ages (see Document 26, p. 86). It was applied especially to bubonic plague during Late Antiquity (the First Pandemic of ca. 540–750 CE) and the Black Death (the name given to the first major outbreak of the Second Pandemic of plague, ca. 1330–1720 CE). Documents 46–48 were written in response to the First Pandemic of bubonic plague (ca. 540–750 CE), often called the Plague of Justinian after the Byzantine emperor (r. 527–65 CE) who contracted and survived the disease. These include accounts of the plague from the Syrian scholar Evagrius Scholasticus (536–94) in Document 46 and Gregory, Bishop of Tours (538–94), in Document 47. Where Evagrius gives a relatively naturalistic description of the symptoms and epidemiology of the plague, Gregory provides a clear example of how the ancient concept of plague as divine punishment did not disappear during the Middle Ages and could exist together with natural explanations.

Document 48 is an explicitly religious reaction to plague (probably bubonic in this case, but the document could be used for any "pestilence"). Throughout the Middle Ages, and to the present day, Catholic priests could perform votive masses for special occasions, which do not correspond to the ordinarily scheduled Divine Office for that day. Special books called *missals* contain instructions and scripts for all kinds of masses, including votive masses. Many missals in northern Europe were influenced by the liturgy and rite performed at Salisbury cathedral in England (also known as Sarum), and the *Sarum Missal* was printed in 1526, which included this votive mass against pestilence. Although this version is later medieval in origin, similar votive masses of healing and protection date back to the early Middle Ages, perhaps the seventh century CE, such as the votive mass of Saint Sigismund to aid those suffering from fever.

Evagrius Scholasticus on the Plague of Justinian[8]

> The Syrian scholar Evagrius Scholasticus (536–94) describes the arrival of the plague in his Greek *Ecclesiastical History*, in which he gives a clear description of the painful swellings, or buboes, typical of bubonic plague. His rhetoric is probably inspired by Thucydides' account of the Plague of Athens in 430 BCE (see Document 9, pp. 35–38), which was a disease other than bubonic plague, but his history is still a valuable source for understanding bubonic plague in the early Middle Ages.

ev

I will also describe the circumstances of the pestilence which commenced at that period, and has now prevailed and extended over the whole world for fifty-two years; a circumstance such as has never before been recorded. Two years after the capture of Antioch by the Persians, a pestilence broke out, in some respects similar to that described by Thucydides, in others widely different. It took its rise from Ethiopia, as is now reported, and made a circuit of the whole world in succession, leaving, as I suppose, no part of the human race unvisited by the disease. Some cities were so severely afflicted as to be altogether depopulated, though in other places the visitation was less violent. It neither commenced according to any fixed period, nor was the time of its cessation uniform; but it seized upon some places at the commencement of winter, others in the course of the spring, others during the summer, and in some cases, when the autumn was advanced. In some instances, having infected a part of a city, it left the remainder untouched; and frequently in an uninfected city one might remark a few households excessively wasted; and in several places, while one or two households utterly perished, the rest of the city remained unvisited: but, as we have learned from careful observation, the uninfected households alone suffered the succeeding year. But the most singular circumstance of all was this; that if it happened that any inhabitants of an infected city were living in a place which the calamity had not visited, these alone were seized with the disorder. This visitation also befell cities and other places in many instances according to the periods called Indictions; and the disease occurred, with the almost utter destruction of human beings, in the second year of each indiction. Thus it happened in my own case—for I deem it fitting, in due adaptation of circumstances, to insert also in this history matters relating

---

8   *The Ecclesiastical History of Evagrius in Six Books* IV.29, translated by E. Walford (London, 1846), 223–26.

to myself—that at the commencement of this calamity I was seized with what are termed **buboes**, while still a school-boy, and lost by its recurrence at different times several of my children, my wife, and many of my kin, as well as of my domestic and country servants; the several indictions making, as it were, a distribution of my misfortunes. Thus, not quite two years before my writing this, being now in the fifty-eighth year of my age, on its fourth visit to Antioch, at the expiration of the fourth indiction from its commencement, I lost a daughter and her son, besides those who had died previously. The plague was a complication of diseases: for, in some cases, commencing in the head, and rendering the eyes bloody and the face swollen, it descended into the throat, and then destroyed the patient. In others, there was a flux of the bowels: in others buboes were formed, followed by violent fever; and the sufferers died at the end of two or three days, equally in possession, with the healthy, of their mental and bodily powers. Others died in a state of delirium, and some by the breaking out of carbuncles. Cases occurred where persons, who had been attacked once and twice and had recovered, died by a subsequent seizure.

The ways in which the disease was communicated, were various and unaccountable: for some perished by merely living with the infected, others by only touching them, others by having entered their chamber, others by frequenting public places. Some, having fled from the infected cities, escaped themselves, but imparted the disease to the healthy. Some were altogether free from contagion, though they had associated with many who were afflicted, and had touched many not only in their sickness but also when dead. Some, too, who were desirous of death, on account of the utter loss of their children and friends, and with this view placed themselves as much as possible in contact with the diseased, were nevertheless not infected; as if the pestilence struggled against their purpose. This calamity has prevailed, as I have already said, to the present time, for two and fifty years, exceeding all that have preceded it. For **Philostratus** expresses wonder that the pestilence which happened in his time, lasted for fifteen years. The sequel is uncertain, since its course will be guided by the good pleasure of God, who knows both the causes of things, and their tendencies. I shall now return to the point from which I digressed, and relate the remainder of Justinian's history.

DOCUMENT 47:

Gregory of Tours on Epidemic Disease and the Sickness of Kings[9]

Like Evagrius Scholasticus (Document 46), the Frankish bishop Gregory of Tours (538–94) also lived through the First Pandemic of plague. He seems to describe that disease in several passages of his Latin *History of the Franks*, but he is not as clear as Evagrius about the symptoms. Gregory names bubonic-like swellings within a list of several diseases that struck the Frankish people because of the sins of their leaders.

e

A very grievous plague followed these prodigies. For while the kings were quarreling and again preparing for civil war, dysentery seized upon nearly the whole of the Gauls. The sufferers had a high fever with vomiting and excessive pain in the kidneys; the head and neck were heavy. Their expectorations were of a saffron color or at least green. It was asserted by many that it was a secret poison. The common people called it internal pimples and this is not incredible, seeing that when cupping glasses were placed on the shoulders or legs **mattery places** formed and broke and the corrupted blood ran out and many were cured. Moreover herbs that are used to cure poisons were drunk and helped a good many. This sickness began in the month of August and seized upon the little ones and laid them on their beds. We lost dear sweet children whom we nursed on our knees or carried in our arms and nourished with attentive care, feeding them with our own hand. But wiping away our tears we say with the blessed Job: "The Lord has given; the Lord has taken away; the Lord's will has been done. Blessed be his name through the ages."

In these days king **Chilperic** was very sick. When he got well his younger son, who was not yet reborn of water and the Holy Spirit, fell ill, and when they saw he was in danger they baptized him. He was doing a little better when his older brother named Clodobert was attacked by the same disease. Their mother Fredegunda saw they were in danger of death and she repented too late, and said to the king: "The divine goodness has long borne with our bad actions; it has often rebuked us with fevers and other evils but repentance did not follow and now we are losing our sons. It is the tears of the poor, the outcries of widows and the sighs of orphans that are destroying them. We have no hope left now in gathering wealth. We get riches and we do not know for whom. Our treasures will be left without

mattery places: Swellings full of diseased matter.

Chilperic: Frankish king of Neustria, r. 561–84.

---

9   Gregory of Tours, *History of the Franks* V.34, translated by Ernest Brehaut (Columbia UP, 1916), 129–30.

an owner, full of violence and curses. Our storehouses are full of wine and our barns of grain, and our treasuries are full of gold, silver, precious stones, necklaces, and all the wealth of rulers. But we are losing what we held more dear. Come, please, let us burn all the wicked tax lists and let what sufficed for your father king Clothar, suffice for your treasury." So the queen spoke, beating her breast with her fists, and she ordered the books to be brought out that had been brought from her cities by Marcus, and when she had thrown them in the fire she said to the king: "Why do you delay; do what you see me do, so that if we have lost our dear children we may at least escape eternal punishment." Then the king repented and burned all the tax books and when they were burned he sent men to stop future taxes. After this the younger child wasted away in great pain and died. They carried him with great grief from Braine to Paris and buried him in the church of St. Denis. Clodobert they placed on a litter and took him to St. Medard's church in Soissons, and threw themselves down at the holy tomb and made vows for him, but being already breathless and weak he died at midnight. They buried him in the holy church of the martyrs Crispin and Crispinian. There was much lamenting among all the people; for men and women followed this funeral sadly wearing the mourning clothes that are customary when a husband or wife dies. After this king Chilperic was generous to cathedrals and churches and the poor.

DOCUMENT 48:

A Votive Mass against Pestilence[10]

This source provides an explicitly religious reaction to plague, a votive mass written to protect its hearers from pestilence. It was written in the later Middle Ages and printed in 1526, but it continues a tradition going back to the Early Middle Ages and the time of the First Pandemic of plague, as seen with Gregory of Tours's religious explanations for plague in Document 47.

ᘓ

A mass to turn away pestilence

Which our lord the Pope Clement composed, and ordained in college with all the cardinals, and he granted to all penitents, truly contrite and confessed, who hear the following mass, two hundred and forty days' **indulgence**. *And all who hear the following mass ought to carry a single burning candle in their hand through the five days following, and to hold it in their hand throughout the whole of the mass, themselves kneeling, and sudden death shall not be able to hurt them. This is certain, and has been proved at Avignon and in the surrounding neighbouring parts.*

Office. Remember thy covenant, O Lord, and say to the destroying angel, Stay now thy hand, that the land be not laid desolate, and that thou destroy not every living soul.
In Easter-tide, Alleluya.

Psalm. Hear, O thou Shepherd of Israel: thou that leadest Joseph like a sheep. [Psalms 80:1]
    Glory be to the Father etc.

Collect. O God, who desirest not the death of a sinner, but rather that he should repent, we beseech thee graciously to convert thy people unto thyself; that whilst they remain devoted unto thee thou mayest mercifully put away from them thy rod of thy wrath. Through etc.

Lesson. [2 Kings 24:15–19] So the Lord sent ... the Lord commanded.

Gradual. The Lord sent his word and healed them: and they were saved from their destruction. [Ps 107:20]

indulgence: In medieval Christianity a religious authority, usually a bishop or the pope, could release a penitent sinner from penance owed (usually measured in days) in exchange for the performance of a specific religious act, such as going on pilgrimage, giving a donation, or hearing a special mass like this one. Indulgences were especially common in times of plague.

---

10 *The Sarum Missal in English*, translated by Frederick E. Warren, 2 vols. (London, 1911–13), Vol. 2, 202–07.

V[erse]. O that men would therefore praise the Lord for his goodness: and declare the wonders that he doeth for the children of men. [Ps 107:21]

Alleluya. *V[erse]*. I will save my people in the midst of Jerusalem, and I will be to them a God in truth and justice. [Zech 8:8]

[Here follows the "Sequence," a lengthy hymn of praise, beseeching God and the Virgin Mary to grant their protection against the plague.]

Gospel. [Luke 4:38–44] And he arose ... synagogues of Galilee.

Offertory. The high-priest stood between the living and the dead, having a golden censer in his hand; and offering the sacrifice of incense he appeased the anger of the Lord, and the plague was stayed from the house and people of Israel. [Numbers 16:46–48]

In Easter-tide, Alleluya.

Secret. We beseech thee, O Lord, that the effect of this present sacrifice may be to succor thy people; that it may mightily save us from all errors and terrors, and guard us and defend us from all assault and loss. Through etc.

Communion. A multitude of diseased, and they that were vexed with unclean spirits, came unto Jesus; for there went virtue out of him, and healed them all. [Luke 6:17–19]

Postcommunion. Hear us, O Lord God of our salvation, and at the intercession of Mary, the blessed mother of God, set thy people free from the terror of thy anger, and of thy mercy make them to rest securely on thy bounty. Through etc.

Sources 49–51 come from one of the most unique and famous episodes in the history of medieval medicine, the flourishing of medicine and medical texts in Anglo-Saxon England (ca. 800–1066 CE). Out of a patchwork of numerous small kingdoms, England gradually unified as a single nation during the ninth and tenth centuries, partly in response to the Danish "Viking" invasions. Alfred the Great, King of Wessex (r. 871–99) is given much of the credit for unifying the Anglo-Saxons politically as well as culturally. This meant encouraging the translation of Latin texts into the Wessex dialect of Old English, including portions of the Bible, writings of St. Augustine and Boethius, as well as medical texts. The *Herbarius* of Apuleius Platonicus (Document 38, pp. 113–15) was translated into Old English and expanded, but the remaining Old English medical texts were new compositions or compilations. These include collections known as the *Lacnunga* (Document 49) and *Bald's Leechbook* (Document 50). The *Lacnunga* is considered a better example of native Anglo-Saxon remedies, in which diseases are personified as elves or evil women, and plants are addressed directly with magical charms invoking both Christ and pagan deities. One example is the famous "Nine Herbs Charm," reproduced in Document 49, in which nine different healing plants are called upon to heal a wide range of diseases and poisons.

While the Old English *Lacnunga* is known best for its magical healing spells, the slightly older *Leechbook* of a physician named Bald reflects the partial incorporation of rational Mediterranean medicine into Anglo-Saxon culture. The remedies in Document 50 are all for eye complaints, and the treatments are entirely natural, without the religious or magical invocations found in the "Nine Herbs Charm" of the *Lacnunga*. The fifth recipe in Document 50, for a wen (a swelling on the eyelid), recently gained fame as the subject of clinical tests by the AncientBiotics Project, an international team of historians of medicine and medical scientists. Their tests suggest that this recipe has valid antibiotic properties against MRSA (Methicillin-resistant Staphylococcus Aureus) bacteria.[11] We must be careful not to use this one example of a medieval recipe that "works" according to our modern criteria as evidence that medieval medicine was "right." The medieval

---

11 "AncientBiotics–a medieval remedy for modern day superbugs?" University of Nottingham Press Release, 30 March 2015. Available at www.nottingham.ac.uk/news/pressreleases/2015/march/ancientbiotics---a-medieval-remedy-for-modern-day-superbugs.aspx.

physicians did not compound, use, or understand these remedies the way we would, and they should be studied in their own historical contexts.

Another type of medical text popular in later Anglo-Saxon England is the *lunarium*, or "moon book," which provides answers to questions based on the day of the month according to the passage of the moon. *Lunaria* provided answers to questions like the following: Should I perform or avoid a certain action? Will my disease intensify or go into remission? Is this a good time to perform bloodletting? What does a lunar eclipse signify for the well-being of my community? Document 51 provides an example of a medical *lunarium*.

DOCUMENT 49:

The *Nine Herbs Charm*, from the Old English *Lacnunga* (tenth century)[12]

Anglo-Saxon England (ca. 800–1066 CE) was the only European culture in the early Middle Ages to produce a significant medical literature in their vernacular language (Old English) rather than in Latin. This literature includes collections known as the *Lacnunga*, excerpted below, and *Bald's Leechbook* (Document 50). The *Lacnunga* is considered a better example of native Anglo-Saxon remedies, in which diseases are personified as elves or evil women, and plants are addressed directly with magical charms invoking both Christ and pagan deities like Woden (Odin). One example is the famous "Nine Herbs Charm" in which nine different healing plants are called upon to heal a wide range of diseases and poisons. There is disagreement over which nine herbs exactly are being described or whether nine are even named in this charm. Most of this source is the charm and the last paragraph provides instructions for how the healer is to use it. Later examples of more fully Christian magico-medical charms are reproduced below in Document 89, pp. 258–59.

❦

"Have a mind, mugwort, what thou mentioned, what thou prepared at the prime telling. 'Una' thou hightest, eldest of **worts**: Thou hast might for three and against thirty, for venom thou availest, for flying vile things; mighty against loathed ones that through the land rove.

And thou, **waybroad**, mother of worts, open from eastward, mighty within; over thee carts creaked, over thee queens rode, over thee brides bridalled, over thee bulls breathed, all these thou withstood, and with attack thou stayed, as thou withstood venom and vile things and all the loathly ones, that through the land rove.

Steem hight this wort, on stone she grew, standeth she gainst venom, stoundeth she attacks head pain. Stiff hight she also, venom she attacks, wreaketh on the wrath one, whirleth out poison.

This is the wort which fought against worm, this avails for venom, for flying vile things. 'Tis good against the loathly ones that through the land rove. Flee now, **attorlothe**, the less from the greater, the greater the less, till boot from them both be.

wort: From *wyrt*, the Old English word for an herb.

waybroad: Also waybread, the Old English name for the common weed plantain.

Steem: watercress.

attorlothe: Identification unknown. Possibly betony or black nightshade. See M.L. Cameron, "What Plant Was Attorlothe (Atorlathe)?" *Parergon* 10:2 (1992), 27–34.

---

12 *Leechdoms, Wortcunning, and Starcraft of Early England* ..., edited and translated by T.O. Cockayne, 3 vols. (London, 1864–66), Vol. 3, 31–39. Some of the text has been modified and modernized because Cockayne invented new words or was intentionally archaic in his translation of the text.

maythen: chamomile.

Alderford: A town in Norfolk, England. It is not clear what chamomile accomplished there.

wergule: crab apple.

Woden: Odin, chief god of the Germanic pantheon, who makes a surprising appearance in this otherwise Christian medical collection.

low it louted: It (the fiend) violently flouted the Lord's command.

watchet: A shade of blue. Most of these "venoms" are distinguished by color.

Have in mind, thou **maythen**, what thou mentioned, what thou accomplished at **Alderford**. That never for flying ill fatally fell man, since we to him maythen for medicine mixed up.

This is the wort which **wergule** hight; this sent the seal over seas ridge of other mischief the malice to mend.

These nine can march on gainst nine ugly poisons. A worm sneaking came to slay and to slaughter; then took up **Woden** nine wondrous twigs, he smote then the adder till it flew in nine bits. There ended it the crab apple and its venom, that never it should more in house come.

Chervil and fennel two fair and mighty ones, these worts the Lord formed, wise he and witty is. Holy in heaven, them he suspended and sent to the seven worlds, for the poor and the rich, Panacea for all. It standeth against pain, it attacks venom, strong it is against three and against thirty; against the hand of the fiend, (to the Lord **low it louted**), against foul fascination of farm stock of mine.

Now these nine worts avail against nine exiles from glory, against nine venoms, and nine flying vile things, against the red venom, against the stinking venom, against the white venom, against the **watchet** venom, against the yellow venom, against the green venom, against the livid venom, against the watchet venom, against the brown venom, against the purple venom, against worm blister, against water blister, against thorn blister, against thistle blister, against ice blister, against poison blister, if any ill come flying from east, or come from north, or any from west, over the human race Christ stood over men opposingly. I alone know Him beaming and the nine adders behold Him. All weeds now may give way to worts. Seas may dissolve, all salt water, when I this venom from thee blow.

Mugwort, waybread which spreadeth open towards the east, cress, attorlothe, maythen, nettle, crab apple, chervil, fennel, and old soap; work the worts to a dust, mingle with the soap and with the verjuice of the apple; form a slop of water and of ashes, take fennel, boil it in the slop, and foment with egg mixture, when the man puts on the salve, either before or after."

Sing the charm upon each of the worts; thrice before he works them up, and over the apple in like manner; and sing into the man's mouth and into both his ears the same magic song, and into the wound, before he applies the salve.

DOCUMENT 50:

Bald's Leechbook: Herbal Remedies for Eye Problems (ninth century)[13]

The *Leechbook* of Bald, written in Old English and Latin, reflects the incorporation of rational Mediterranean medicine into Anglo-Saxon culture. The remedies translated below are all for eye complaints, and the treatments are entirely natural, without the religious or magical invocations found in the "Nine Herbs Charm" of the *Lacnunga* above (Document 49).

＊＊＊

For much eye ache. Many a man hath much ache in his eyes. Work him then groundsel and bishopwort and fennel, boil all the worts in water, milk is better, make that throw up a reek on the eyes. Again, let him mingle with wine celandine and woodbine leaves and the herb cuckoo-sour.

Again for much eye ache pound in wine the nether part of cropleek and the nether part of Wihtmars wort, let it stand two days. For **pearl**, an eye salve; take ashes of broom and a bowl full of hot wine, pour this by a little at a time thrice on the hot ashes, and put that then into a brass or a copper vessel, add somewhat of honey and mix together, apply to the infirm man's eyes, and again wash the eyes in a clean well spring. For pearl on the eye, apply the gall of a hare, warm, for about two days, it flieth from the eyes. Against the white spot, mingle together vinegar and burnt salt and barley meal, apply it to the eye, hold thine hand a long while on it.

For pearl, an eye salve; take seed of celandine or the root of it, rub it into old wine and into honey, add pepper, let it stand for a night by the fire, use it when thou wilt sleep. Against white spot, boil in butter the nether part of ox-slip and alder rind.

In case the eyes be tearful, juice of rue, and goat's gall and bumblebee honey, of all equal quantities. If eyes be tearful, add to sweetened wine ashes of hart's horn.

Work an eye salve for a wen, take cropleek and garlic, of both equal quantities, pound them well together, take wine and bullock's gall, of both equal quantities, mix with the leek, put this then into a brazen vessel, let it stand nine days in the brass vessel, wring out through a cloth and clear it well, put it into a horn, and about night time apply it with a feather to the eye; the best leechdom.

For a wen on the eye, take hollow cress, roast it, apply it to the eye, as hot as possible.

pearl: An eyelid infection that apparently looks round and white, probably a chalazion.

---

13   *Leechdoms, Wortcunning, and Starcraft*, Vol. 2, 33–37. Modified.

For eye ache, let him work for himself groundsel and bishopwort and beewort and fennel, boil all the worts in water; milk is better.

For ache of eyes, take the red hove, boil it in sour beer or in sour ale, and bathe the eyes in the bath, the oftener the better.

For eye ache, take twigs of withewind, pound them, boil them in butter, apply them to the eyes.

Work an eye salve thus; take nut kernels and wheat grains, rub them together, add wine, strain through a cloth, then apply to the eyes. For acute pain and ache of eyes, mingle well crumbs of white bread and pepper and vinegar, lay this on a cloth, bind it on the eyes for a night. Thus shall a man work an eye salve, take the nether part of strawberry plants and pepper, pound them well, put them on a cloth, bind them fast, lay them in sweetened wine, make somebody drop one drop into the eyes. Work an eye salve thus; leaves of woodbine, woodmarch, strawberry plants, southern wormwood, green hellebore, celandine, pound the worts much, mingle with wine, put into a copper vessel or keep in a brazen vat, let it stand seven days or more, wring the worts very clean, add pepper, and sweeten very lightly with honey, put subsequently into a horn, and with a feather put one drop into the eyes.

DOCUMENT 51:

Medical Prognostics in Anglo-Saxon England[14]

A *lunarium* was a medieval text used for determining future events based on phases of the moon or days of the month. *Lunaria* provide a simple example of medieval astrology, based on the belief that the moon and other celestial bodies influenced our bodies and actions. Some *lunaria*, like the one below, were medical in nature and provide a simple prognosis according to what day of the month the patient fell ill. This medical *lunarium* was written originally in Latin and comes from a famous Anglo-Saxon manuscript known as Cotton Tiberius A.III, now in the British Library. The manuscript contains 20 different prognostic texts, including this one, written in Latin, Anglo-Saxon, or both. Only a few prognostics are explicitly medical; others describe the meaning of dreams, the significance of thunder, weather forecasts, and other omens.

e

1. Whoever falls sick on the first day of the month will escape with difficulty.
2. The second day of the month, he will quickly rise again.
3. The third day of the month, he will not escape.
4. The fourth day of the month, he will struggle and arise.
5. The fifth day of the month, he will sink and arise.
6. The sixth day of the month, he will not escape.
7. The seventh day of the month, he will be healed with medicine.
8. The eighth day of the month, he will suffer long, then arise.
9. The ninth day of the month, he will languish.
10. The tenth day of the month, he will be sick for a long time.
11. The eleventh day of the month, he will be threatened by danger.
12. The twelfth day of the month, he will arise.
13. The thirteenth day of the month, he will be sick for a certain time.
14. The fourteenth day of the month, he will struggle and arise.
15. The fifteenth day of the month, he will be in danger.
16. The sixteenth day of the month, he will change his place, and arise.
17. The seventeenth day of the month, he will sink and arise.
18. The eighteenth day of the month, he will struggle and arise.
19. The nineteenth day of the month, likewise.
20. The twentieth day of the month, likewise.

---

14 R.M. Liuzza, *Anglo-Saxon Prognostics: An Edition and Translation of Texts from London, British Library, MS Cotton Tiberius A.III* (D.S. Brewer, 2011), 165, 167, 169, 201.

21. The twenty-first day of the month, he will help the thing.
22. The twenty-second day of the month, he will languish and arise.
23. The twenty-third day of the month, likewise.
24. The twenty-fourth day of the month, he will languish for a long time.
25. The twenty-fifth day of the month, he will languish and die.
26. The twenty-sixth day of the month, he will languish.
27. The twenty-seventh day of the month, he will sink and arise.
28. The twenty-eighth day of the month, a sick man will lie for a long time, then die.
29. The twenty-ninth day of the month, a sick man will escape.
30. The thirtieth day of the month, a sick man will struggle, and arise.

PART 7

The Arabic Tradition of Learned Medicine (ca. 900–1400 CE)

In the centuries after the death of Galen (ca. 210 CE), his medical writings were widely accepted as the basis of a proper medical education. This was especially true in the Eastern half of the Roman Empire, where education of all kinds continued even after the loss of the Western Roman Empire in 476 CE, and where many people could still read Greek. Scholars in Alexandria (like Paul of Aegina, Document 40, pp. 118–19), which had been an important medical center since the Hellenistic period, developed a formal medical curriculum based on about twenty of Galen's works. This Galenic corpus remained the foundation of Greek and Islamicate medical education for the rest of the Middle Ages.[1] Alexandria, however, and much of the Eastern Roman Empire, were conquered by the new Islamic caliphate in the seventh century CE. After Islamic political control of North Africa and the Middle East was settled, the Muslim leaders allowed and encouraged the translation of Greek science, philosophy, and medicine into Arabic. This occurred not in Alexandria, but primarily at the Abbasid Islamic capital at Baghdad, and through this translation movement, medicine in the Islamicate world became thoroughly Galenic.

One of the most prolific translators in Baghdad was an Arab Christian physician and scholar named Hunayn ibn Ishaq (809–73 CE). He wrote and translated many works, but his most famous was a brief summary of Galenic medicine called "Questions on Medicine" (Document 52). This work was translated from Arabic into Latin during the later eleventh century by a Christian monk from Kairouan (modern Tunisia) known as Constantine the African (see Document 62, pp. 188–90 and Document 66, pp. 199–200). Hunayn came to be known as Johannitius in Latin Europe and his "Questions of Medicine" were renamed the *Isagoge* (Greek for "Introduction"). By the early twelfth century in Europe, the *Isagoge* and several other Hippocratic and Galenic works were organized into a set

---

1   A.Z. Iskandar, "An Attempted Reconstruction of the Late Alexandrian Medical Curriculum," *Medical History* 20:3 (1976), 235–58.

curriculum, known as the *Art of Medicine* and later as the *Articella* ("little art"), used for teaching the basics of scholarly medicine.

The *Isagoge* of Johannitius was read and taught for centuries as an accessible introduction to medical theory. Medieval physicians looking for much more information on medical theory and practice as well could turn to the medical encyclopedia *al-Qānūn fī al-Tibb*, or *The Canon of Medicine*, of Avicenna (Document 53). Avicenna (Ibn Sīnā, 980–1037), was a Persian-Arabic physician and arguably the most important author for the study of medicine in the later Middle Ages, not only in the Islamicate world, but also in Christian Europe after the translation of his works into Latin during the twelfth and thirteenth centuries. A true polymath, Avicenna composed many treatises on medicine, law, mathematics, physics, and philosophy. Avicenna also wrote a summary of medicine in Arabic verse called *al-'Arjuzat fi't-tibb* (also *'Urguza fi't-Tibb*), known in Latin Europe as *Cantica Avicennae* (Document 54). Reproduced in Document 54 is Avicenna's section on diagnosis by studying the patient's urine, known as uroscopy or urinalysis. Through the influence of Avicenna and other Arabic physicians, urinalysis became one of the most common practices of learned physicians everywhere in Europe and the Mediterranean for centuries to come.

Many physicians and medical authors in the Islamicate world were not Muslims, but Jews. The best known was Moses Maimonides (1135/1138–1204), the Greek name of Rabbi Moshe ben Maimon, a Spanish Sephardic Jew and an accomplished author in both Hebrew and Arabic. He is revered to this day among Jews as "RAMBAM" (an acronym of his Hebrew name), thanks to his 14-volume *Mishneh Torah*, an extensive theological and philosophical commentary on the Hebrew Bible and Talmud. But he was renowned around the medieval Mediterranean as an astronomer and physician, and at least 10 of his medical works survive. Maimonides wrote these secular works in Judeo-Arabic (Arabic written with Hebrew letters), because he lived his entire life in the predominantly Arabic and Islamic cities of Córdoba and Cairo. He was a close reader of the works of Galen and Hippocrates, which he knew in Arabic translations, as demonstrated in his *Commentary on Hippocrates' Aphorisms* and *Abridgements of the Works of Galen*. He also wrote specific treatises on asthma, poison, sexual intercourse, hemorrhoids, and drugs. His most famous and longest medical work was his *Medical Aphorisms*, drawn primarily from Galen's writings. Though not wholly original, the *Medical Aphorisms* (Document 55) have the great value of rationally summarizing and thematically organizing many of the diverse ideas scattered in Galen's voluminous writings.

Abū Bakr Muhammad ibn Zakariyyā al-Rāzī (ca. 865–925 CE), or "Rhazes" as he was known in Europe was a physician from Tehran, working in Baghdad, and trained in Arabic-Galenic medicine. Al-Rāzī supposedly wrote more than 200 books, mostly on medicine and pharmacy, but also on philosophy and music. Two of his most popular works were medical encyclopedias, both translated into Latin, and known in Europe as the *Liber ad Almansorem* ("The Book for al-Mansur") and the *Liber Continens* (named after its first word in the Latin translation, *continens*, "containing"). While those lengthy works are primarily composed of excerpts from ancient authors like Hippocrates, Galen, and Oribasius, one of his works is a collection of case studies, which seem to come directly from a notebook of patient observations, loosely arranged into a single treatise (Document 56). They are similar to the case studies from the Hippocratic *Epidemics* (Document 12, pp. 46–48), and the two sets were to be read together and compared, as al-Rāzī himself says.

Al-Rāzī displays a positive model of his own interactions with patients, but another Arabic author, Usamah ibn Munqidh (1095–1188 CE), provides both negative and positive models through his observation of contemporary physicians. In one passage of his *Memoirs* (Document 57) Usamah describes the medical practice of "Frankish" (that is, Western European Christian) doctors in the Crusader states. All European invaders or pilgrims were called *Franj* (Franks) in Arabic. Although not a physician himself, Usamah provides valuable comparisons between European and Islamicate medical practice in the twelfth century.

Al-Rāzī also wrote the *Kitab al-Jadari wa-al-Hasba*, or "Book on Smallpox and Measles," which demonstrates a willingness to break with the past (Document 58). This work holds an important place in the history of medicine, as one of the first works to demonstrate what is now called "differential diagnosis" to identify and distinguish between diseases in a patient (in this case, smallpox and measles). The "Book on Smallpox and Measles" is an excellent example of how a learned, medieval physician could move beyond the teachings of Galen, while still holding him in high esteem. The book is organized into 14 chapters, following a pattern typical of Arabic and Latin medieval authors, reviewing what the ancients said, detailing the theory of the disease, then describing practical treatments.

One of the most important acts of devotion for Muslims is to make a pilgrimage, or *hajj*, to the city of Mecca, now in Saudi Arabia. For many medieval Muslims, this journey was long and arduous, and intended for penance and devotion. Even though a pilgrimage is supposed to be difficult, one Arabic Christian physician and scientist, Qustā ibn Lūqā (820–912 CE), sought to ease the pilgrims' journey by compiling a health guide for them, *Medical Regime for the Pilgrims at Mecca* (Document 59), the only known example of this sort of work. He treats a variety of subjects related to the health and well-being of travelers, but this work is especially remarkable for his extended discussion of guinea worm disease (dracunculiasis), an infection caused by the parasitic nematode *Dracunculus medinensis*. Some of Qustā's medical and philosophical treatises (although not this one) were later translated into Latin, and Europeans knew him as "Costa ben Luca."

After the Islamic conquests of the former Eastern Roman Empire during the seventh and eighth centuries CE, the Muslim elites incorporated much of ancient Greco-Roman medicine and philosophy into their culture. Muslim medical authors sought to balance the teachings of the Prophet with those of Galen and Hippocrates, much as Jewish and Christian authors had sought a balance between biblical revelation and Greco-Roman ("pagan") philosophy. Al-Suyūtī (ca. 1445–1505 CE) was an Egyptian religious scholar and prolific author of commentaries on the Quran. His book *'Al-Tibb al-Nabawī* (Document 60) records centuries of scholarship on the "Medicine of the Prophet" and combines it with teachings of ancient Greek and medieval Islamicate rational physicians.

Hunayn ibn Ishaq's Introduction to Rational Medicine[2]

Hunayn ibn Ishaq (809–73 CE), known as Johannitius in Latin Europe, was an Arab Christian physician and scholar in Baghdad. Of his many medical treatises and translations, his most famous is a brief summary of Galenic medicine called "Questions on Medicine." In this work he outlines the humors, elements, qualities, and other aspects of the human body and health. Most importantly for the development of medieval medicine, he described succinctly several defining aspects of medieval medicine which were not original to Galen, but had been synthesized from his works by later Alexandrian and Arabic scholars: the "naturals" (defining aspects of the human body including the humors and elements), "non-naturals" (external influences which affect health such as exercise, baths, food, drink, sleep, sexual activity, and emotions), and "contra-naturals" (diseases and aging).

∾

The Beginning of the Introduction of Johannitius to Medicine

Medicine is divided into two parts, namely theoretical and practical. And of these two the theoretical is further divided into three, that is to say, the consideration of the naturals, the non-naturals, and the contra-naturals. From the consideration of these arises the knowledge of sickness, of health, and of the mean state, and their causes and significations; of when the four humors increase in an abnormal manner, or of what may be the cause or significance of sickness.

Of the Naturals. The naturals are seven in number: elements, qualities, humors, members, energies, operations, and **spirits**. But some add to these four others: namely, age, color, figure, and the distinction between male and female.

The Elements. There are four elements: fire, air, water, and earth. Fire is hot and dry; air is hot and moist; water is cold and moist; earth is cold and dry.

The Qualities. There are nine qualities, eight unequal and one equal. Of the unequal, four are simple: namely, hot, cold, moist, and dry. From these arise four compound qualities: hot and moist, hot and dry, cold and moist, cold and dry. The equal is when the body is so disposed that it is in good condition and in a mean state, when it has a proper amount of all four.

spirits: Intangible life forces which course through the body, not to be confused with the soul in the monotheist traditions.

2   Johannitius, *Isagoge*, in *John of Gaddesden and the Rosa Medicinae*, translated by H.P. Cholmeley (Oxford, 1912), 136–66, with minor changes to spelling and punctuation.

Of the Humors. The humors are four in number: namely, blood, phlegm, reddish bile, and black bile. Blood is hot and moist, phlegm is cold and moist, reddish bile is hot and dry, black bile is cold and dry.

Of phlegm. There are five varieties of phlegm. There is the salt phlegm, which is hotter and drier than the rest and is tinged with the biliary humor. There is the sweet phlegm belonging to hotness and dampness, which is tinged with the sanguine humor. There is the acrid phlegm belonging to coldness and dryness, which is tinged with the melancholic humor. There is the glassy phlegm, which arises from great coldness and coagulation such as occurs in old people who are destitute of natural warmth. And there is another which is cold and moist; it has no odor, but retains its own coldness and moistness.

Of reddish bile. Reddish bile exists in five different fashions. There is reddish bile which is clear or pure and hot, both by nature and substance, of which the origin is from the liver. There is another which is straw-colored, from which the origin is from the watery humor of phlegm, and pure reddish bile, and therefore it is less hot. Another is vitelline. It is similar to the yolk of an egg, and it has its origin from a mixture of coagulated phlegm and clear red bile, like the green of a leek, and it arises generally from the stomach or the liver; and there is another which is green like verdigris, and which burns after the fashion of a poison, and its origin is from too much **adustio**, and it possesses its own proper color and its own energies, both good and evil.

Of black bile. Black bile exists in two different fashions. In one way it may be said to be natural to the dregs of blood and any disturbance of the same, and it can be known from its black color whether it flows out of the body from below or above, and its property is cold and dry. The other kind is altogether outside the course of nature, and its origin is from the *adustio* of the **choleric** quality, and so it is rightly called black, and it is hotter and lighter, and having in itself a most deadly quality and a pernicious character.

[Johannitius continues to enumerate the four primary organs of the body, the three energies, two operations, three spirits, four ages, then skin color, hair color, and parts of the eye.]

Of the Qualities of the Body. The qualities of the body are five in number: namely, excess or grossness; thinness or tenuity; wasting, squalidity, and the mean state. There are two kinds of grossness, the one consisting in excess of flesh, and the other in fat. Excess of flesh arises from excess of heat and humors; but fatness from cold and intense humidity; loss of fat or thinness arises from heat and intense dryness. Wasting arises from cold and intense humidity, or from an intensity of both together. And the mean state arises from a proper proportion of the humors. These are the appearances of the body.

adustio: The harmful burning or scorching of a humor, usually by fever.

choleric: Relating to yellow bile, *cholera,* and to anger, the emotion which was believed to be provoked by an excess of it.

Of the Difference between Male and Female. The male differs from the female in that he is hotter and more dry; she, on the contrary, is colder and more moist.

The Beginning of the Treatise on the Non-naturals

And first of the Changes of the air. Changes of the air come about in five different ways; from the seasons, from the rising and setting of the stars, from the winds, and from the different countries and their exhalations.

Of the seasons. There are four seasons; namely, Spring, which is hot and moist; Summer, which is hot and dry; Autumn, which is cold and dry; Winter, which is cold and moist. The nature of the air is also changed by the stars, for when the sun approaches a star or a star the sun, the air becomes hotter. But when they separate, the coldness of the air is altered, namely, either increased or diminished.

Of the Number and Properties of the Winds. There are four winds; the East, the West, the North, and the South. And of these the nature of one is cold and dry and of another hot and moist. The two others are of an equal nature, for the East is hot and dry and the West is cold and moist. The South is slightly hotter and moister and the North colder and dryer.

Of Varieties of Places and their Qualities. There are four varieties of places; namely, height, depth, nearness to mountains or to the sea, and those particular qualities in which one district differs from another. Height produces cold and depth the contrary. The relation to mountains is as follows: if the mountains are to the south, the locality will be the cooler, for the mountains keep off the hot winds, and so the north winds seek it out with their cool breath. But if the mountains are to the north of the locality the reverse is the case. As regards relation to the sea: if the sea is on the south the locality will be hot and dry, if to the north it will be cold and dry. Soils differ among themselves. Stony land is cold and dry; fat and heavy land is hot and moist; clay lands are cold and moist. Exhalations from marshy land or other places where decay is going on also change the air and give rise to disease and pestilence.

[Johannitius then enumerates the non-naturals, including exercise, baths, food, drink, sleep, sexual activity, and emotions, what were called "affections" or "accidents" of the mind.]

Of the Contra-naturals

There are three contra-naturals; namely, disease, the cause of disease, and the concomitants or sequel of disease. Disease is that which primarily injures the body, without the aid of any intermediary, as, for instance, heat in continuous fever.

Of Fevers. Fever is an unnatural heat, i.e. heat which overpasses the normal course of nature. And it proceeds from the heart into the arteries, and is harmful by its own effects. And of it there are three kinds: the first in the spirit, which is called ephemeral; the second arises from the humors which putrefy, and which is therefore called putrid; and the third affects for ill the solid portions of the body, and this is called **hectic**. Of these three the ephemeral variety arises from non-essential causes.

Putrid fever arises from putrid matters, and these are simple and uncombined, and they are four in number. The first is that which arises from putridity of the blood and burns up both the interior and exterior of the body; such, for instance, is continuous fever. The second is that which arises from putridity of reddish bile; such, for instance, is tertian fever. The third arises from putridity of phlegm; such, for instance, is quotidian fever. And the fourth arises from putridity of black bile; this attacks the sick man after an interval of two days, and it is called quartan.

In addition there are three kinds of fevers occurring from putridity. First there is the fever which lessens day by day; such, for instance, as that called *peraugmasticus*, i.e. decreasing. Secondly, that which increases until it departs; such as that called *augmasticus*. Thirdly, that which neither decreases nor increases until it again departs; such, for instance, as that called *homothenus*.

Continued fever arising from putridity in the veins begins to decline by departing from out the veins into other parts of the body. Goose-skin or shivering occurs in fevers from an infusion of putrid matter in to the sensitive members, which gnaws and makes them cold. And, therefore, goose-skin occurs in these fevers which are characterized by remissions or variations, for the putrid matters are outside the veins....

Of the Qualities of the Body. The qualities of the body are three in number: namely, health, sickness, and the mean state. Health is that condition in which the temperament of the body and the seven naturals are working according to the course of nature. Sickness is defect in temperament outside the course of nature, and injuring nature, whence arises an effect of harm which may be felt. The mean state is that which is neither health nor disease. And there are three kinds of this mean state: (*a*) when health and disease co-exist in the same body; which may happen in different members, as in the blind or the lame; (*b*) in the bodies of the aged, in whom no one member remains that is not in evil case or suffers; (*c*) in those who are well at one season and sick at another. For instance, persons of a cold nature are sick in the winter and well in the summer; and those of a moist nature are sick in childhood, but well in youth and old age. Those of a dry nature are well in childhood, but sick in youth and old age.

hectic: The term is still used occasionally for intermittent, violent fevers, but here Hunayn (Johannitius) uses it to refer to fevers arising from the corruption of the solid portions of the body.

Health, sickness, and the mean state are evident in three ways; (1) in the body in which any one of them occurs; (2) in the cause which produces, which governs, and which preserves them; (3) in their indicating signs....

Of the Regimen of Health. The regimen of health is of three kinds according as it deals with those prone to illness, those just beginning to be ill, and weakly persons. The first classes are treated by proper regulation of the aforesaid six things, i.e. the non-naturals. Those in the second class are treated in two ways; first, by removal of the excess of humor; secondly, by repairing any defect in nature and by counseling adherence to the proper observance of the non-naturals. "Weakly persons" are infants, old persons, and convalescents.

Avicenna, *The Canon of Medicine*[3]

The Persian-Arabic physician Avicenna (Ibn Sīnā, 980–1037) is best known for his massive medical encyclopedia *al-Qānūn fī al-Tibb*, or *The Canon of Medicine*. According to the legends that accrued around him, he composed this work when he was only 21 years old. The Greek *kanón*, Latin *canon*, and Arabic *qānūn* are all cognate words, meaning a "law" or "standard," and Avicenna's *Canon* became the standard against which all learned medicine among Christians, Jews, and Muslims came to be measured. He provided a clear and organized synthesis of the medical teachings of Hippocrates, Galen, Dioscorides, and Late Antique physicians from the Latin, Greek, Syrian, and Persian traditions. The *Canon* is still used today in parts of southwest Asia and India as the foundation of *Unani* medicine which blends the Hippocratic humoralism with elements from Persian, Indian, and Chinese traditional medicines. Gerard of Cremona translated the *Canon* into Latin in the later twelfth century, and during the thirteenth century it became a foundational text for teaching medicine in European universities.

The *Canon* contains five lengthy books: 1) general medical principles, 2) pharmaceuticals, 3) pathology and treatment of diseases in individual organs (organized head to toe), 4) medical conditions of the whole body (fevers and poisons), and 5) a "formulary" of over 600 medicinal compounds and their uses. Because of its massive size, the *Canon* rarely circulated as a complete text in Arabic or Latin. Instead, individual books, or parts of books, were copied and circulated, along with commentaries by later teachers and readers. The selections in Document 53 come from Book 1 of the *Canon* (on general medical principles), which Avicenna divided according to logical principles into twenty-five "lectures." These lectures are organized into five parts: 1.1) the material basis of medicine and disease, 1.2) the causes of disease, 1.3) the symptoms of disease, 1.4) the preservation of health, and 1.5) therapeutics. These selections demonstrate Avicenna's rigorously logical exposition of how the human body, its parts, and its functions are derived from the four elements, the four humors, and their four qualities.

---

3   Avicenna, *The Canon of Medicine (al-Qānūn fi'l-tibb)*, adapted by Laleh Bakhtiar, from the translation of Vol. 1 by O. Cameron Gruner and Mazhar H. Shah, correlated with the Arabic by Jay R. Crook, with notes by O. Cameron Gruner (KAZI Publication, 1999), 9, 11, 15, 17–18, 31–32, 45. Punctuation modified.

Lecture 1: The Scope of Medicine and Its Topics

Medicine is the science by which we learn the various states of the human body in health and when not in health, and the means by which health is likely to be lost and, when lost, is likely to be restored back to health. In other words, it is the art whereby health is conserved and the art whereby it is restored after being lost....

Medicine deals with the states of health and disease in the human body. It is a truism of philosophy that a complete knowledge of a thing can only be obtained by elucidating its causes and antecedents, provided, of course, such causes exist. In medicine it is, therefore, necessary that causes of both health and disease should be determined.

Sometimes these causes are obvious to the senses but at other times they may defy direct observation. In such circumstances, causes and antecedents have to be carefully inferred from the signs and symptoms of the disease. Hence, a description of the signs and symptoms of disease is also necessary for our purpose. It is a dictum of the exact sciences that knowledge of a thing is attained only through a knowledge of the causes and origins of the causes—assuming there to be causes and origins. Consequently our knowledge cannot be complete without an understanding both of symptoms and of the principles of being....

Lecture 2: The Elements

The elements are simple substances which are the primary constituents of the human body and which cannot be subdivided into further ingredients. It is by their combination and appropriate organization that the various orders of things in nature have been formed. Natural philosophy speaks of four elements and no more. Two of these are light and two heavy. Fire and air are light while earth and water are heavy....

Lecture 3: The Temperaments

Temperament is the quality which results from the mutual interaction of the four contrary, primary qualities of elements. By dividing up into minute particles, the elements are able to secure an intimate contact among themselves. These elements are so minutely intermingled as each to lie in very intimate relationship to one another. Their opposite powers alternately conquer and become conquered until a state of equilibrium is reached which is uniform throughout the whole. It is this outcome that is called "the temperament." Since the primary powers in the elements are four in number (namely: heat, cold, moisture, dryness), it is evident that the temperaments in bodies undergoing generation and destruction accord with these powers. A simple, rational classification is of two types: (a) Equable or balanced. Here the contrary qualities are present to exactly equal degrees of potency—neither of them being in excess or deficiency. This temperament has a quality which is exactly the mean between the two extremes. (b) Inequable or unbalanced. Here the quality of the temperament is not an exquisitely exact mean between the two contraries, but tends a little more to one than to the other. For example, to hot more than to cold; to moist more than to dry; or contrariwise.

It is to be noted that a temperament, as understood by medicine, is never strictly equable or strictly inequable. The physician should abide by the philosopher, who is aware that the really "equable" temperament does not actually exist in the human being any more than it exists in any "member" or "organ." Moreover, the term "equable," used by doctors in their treatises does not refer to weight but to an equity of distribution. It is this distribution which is the primary consideration—whether one is referring to the body as a whole, or only to some individual member; and the average measure of the elements in it, as to quantity and quality, is that which standard human nature ought to have—both in best proportion and in equity of distribution. As a matter of fact, the mean between excess and deficiency of qualities, such as is characteristic of man, actually is very close to the theoretical ideal....

Lecture 4: The Humors

Humor or body-fluid is that fluid, moist, physical substance into which our aliment is transformed. That part of the aliment which has the capacity to be transformed into body substance, either by itself or in combination with something else thereby being capable of assimilation by the members or organs, and completely integrated into the tissues, is the healthy or good humor. It is what replaces the loss which the body substance undergoes.

The residue from the process, the "superfluity," is called unhealthy or abnormal humor. It is this fluid which, in the absence of proper digestion or conversion, is unsuitable for assimilation and is therefore eliminated from the body.

Body fluids may be primary or secondary. Primary fluids are the sanguineous humor (blood), the serous humor (phlegm), the bilious humor (yellow bile) and the atrabilious humor (black bile). Secondary fluids of the body are either non-excrements or excrements. The non-excrements have not yet been subjected to any action by any of the simple organs and they are not changed until they reach the destined tissues. They are of four types: (1) that which is located at the orifices of the minutest channels near the tissues and thus irrigating them; (2) that which permeates the tissues like a dew and is capable of being transformed into nutriment if it becomes necessary; (3) the third type forms a nutrient which will be changed into the substance of the tissues, whether to the extent of entering into their temperament or to the extent of changing into their very essence, thereby attaining an entire likeness to the member or organ. (4) The fourth type accounts for the continuous identity of the member or organ or of the body throughout one's life. It is derived from the semen, which in its turn is derived from the humors.

The non-excreted fluids have not as yet been subjected to the action of any of the simple members or organs and they are to be changed until they reach the tissues for which they are destined. The second type mentioned above—the fluid which is present in the tissues as dew drops and is capable of being utilized as a nutriment in times of dire necessity, also moistens the organs which have been dried up by excessive activity....

Avicenna on Prognosis through Urine[4]

Avicenna wrote a summary of medicine in Arabic verse called *al-'Arjuzat fi't-tibb*, known in Latin as *Cantica Avicennae* ("Song of Avicenna"). The *Cantica* gives us a good indication of the general shape of Islamicate medical education in the central Middle Ages. In the later thirteenth century, perhaps around 1284, a physician in Montpellier named Armengaud de Blaise translated Avicenna's poem into Latin prose. Avicenna's *Poem* is vastly shorter than his *Canon* (Document 53), but he still attempted to include all necessary aspects of medicine within it. The work is divided into two parts, one on medical theory and one on medical practice. The first section is devoted to medical theory and is organized much like the *Isagoge* of Hunayn ibn Ishaq (Document 52). The second, practical section of the *Poem* is divided into two lengthy chapters. One is on the maintenance of health through diet and drugs, and the other is on returning the patient to health through the same dietary regimen and drugs. Almost as an afterthought, Avicenna adds a much shorter section on surgical practice with three "chapters" of only a few lines each, on bloodletting, surgery, and setting bones. Reproduced here is Avicenna's section on diagnosis by studying the patient's urine, known as uroscopy or urinalysis.

e

Symptoms Obtained from the Function of the Liver

It is in the liver that the humors are born; from there they are spread throughout the body. Every organ functions because of it and it alone has no need of the others. The vital spirit is born in the vapor of the liver; the body is healthy according to its state. If the humors are healthy, the body is; the former are if the liver is in good state. Water carries food to it and the water is mixed with the predominant humor and, with its expulsion in the urine, shows that it contained residues. Urine has different colors and everything that the humors have left in it appears to us as a sediment. It is apparent, from what I have stated and wise men witness it, that urine is a faithful guide for the knowledge of the illness.

---

4   Haven C. Krueger, *Avicenna's Poem on Medicine* (Charles C. Thomas, Publisher, 1963), 36–39.

On Urine and First about the Color

While urine witnesses the quantity of ingested food and drink, it is a sign of bad digestion, phlegm, cold, restlessness or of **hepatic** obstruction. Somewhat yellow, it indicates the presence of a certain quantity of bile. The color of fire, that means the presence of a great deal of yellow bile. Very yellow and tinted with red, it proves a superabundance of yellow bile. Dark red urine of the one who has ingested **saffron** and who has had neither fever nor colic contains blood. When found black after having been dark, it signifies that the patient has suffered a great chill. Black after having been very red indicates a poor combustion of humors. Judge the illness according to the odor of urine on the condition that the patient has not ingested a coloring food, certain vegetables, **cassia fistula** and that which may tint like **murri**.

hepatic: Related to the liver.

saffron: The spice saffron produces a deep orange color in food and urine.

cassia fistula: Dried fruits from a tree related to cinnamon.
murri: A condiment made of fermented barley by medieval Greeks and Arabs.

On the Density of Urine

The tenuity of the urine indicates inadequacy of digestion. Sometimes it is fluid after indigestion or obstruction of the liver or because of a tumor. The thickness of the urine indicates good digestion or the abundance of phlegm in the body.

On the Sediments in Urine

The white sediment indicates recovery; yellow, it marks acuteness of the bile; if it is red like the bloodwort, it is a question of disease of the blood. If a similar sediment continues without modification, that indicates an abscess of the liver. Black after having been dark red and that after loss of strength, going to the bottom after having floated, that means the soul is about to escape; the patient can no longer benefit from the prayers of a sorcerer; death is at hand through the excess humoral combustion. If the sediment appears black after having been dark and if it does not occur in the course of an acute illness, especially if this appearance coincides with a favorable sign, and if the origin of the illness is in black bile, it indicates the end of the illness.

On the Location of the Sediment

If a cloud appears floating in the upper portion of the vial, it indicates crudeness of the illness. If a certain maturity exists in the urine, **wind** is causing the sediment to reascend to the surface. If the sediment is half-way up, be aware that the wind is in small quantity. If it is white, after having been

wind: Here this probably means gassiness or "wind" in the patient.

yellow, coherent without being thick, falls to the bottom, appears with a changeable color, it marks the maturity of the illness.

On the Consistency of the Sediment

An ephemeral sediment indicates the weakness of the patient. If there are elements similar to barley meal in the urine, one is dealing with scrapings of the vessels. If the sediment looks like bran and has a bad odor, it indicates ulceration within the ducts; like metal filings, it proves the elimination of portions of organs. If pus appears in the vial, it marks the opening of a collection. If the sediment has decomposed blood, there is a **phlegmonous tumor**. If it goes to the bottom, resembles sperm, it comes from an immature lymph swelling. If one sees sand in it, be aware that there is a **calculus**.

phlegmonous tumor: A swelling judged to be full of the humor phlegm.

calculus: A kidney or bladder stone.

On the Odor of Urine

If the urine has no odor, it is that the food has not been digested or has been ingested raw. The degree of decomposition agrees with the intensity of the odor of the urine. If this odor is dreadful, be aware that the illness is in the bladder. Thus, I have reported on the different kinds of urine; guide yourself by what I have stated about their composition.

DOCUMENT 55:
Maimonides and Galen on the Meaning of the Pulse[5]

> Moses Maimonides (1135/1138–1204 CE) was a Spanish Sephardic Jew and
> an accomplished author in both Hebrew and Judeo-Arabic (Arabic written
> with Hebrew letters). He used Hebrew for his Jewish theological writings
> and Judeo-Arabic for his non-religious books on astronomy and medicine.
> His longest medical work was *Medical Aphorisms*, a compilation in 25 books
> of about 1,500 pithy statements, or aphorisms, drawn primarily from Galen's
> writings. The excerpts below come from Maimonides' summary of Galen's
> aphorisms about reading a patient's pulse. Next to the analysis of urine
> (uroscopy), pulse reading became one of the most important diagnostic tools
> for learned physicians throughout the medieval world. Maimonides explains
> in his prologue his methods for choosing and organizing these Hippocratic-
> Galenic ideas about the pulse.

e

[Prologue]

... I do not claim to have authored these aphorisms that I have set down in
writing. I would rather say that I have selected them—that is, I have selected
them from Galen's words from all his books, both from his original works
and from his commentaries to the books of Hippocrates. In these aphorisms
I have not adhered to the method that I followed in the *Epitomes*, in which I
quoted Galen's very words, as I stipulated in the introduction to the *Epitomes*.
Rather, most of the aphorisms that I have selected are in the very words of
Galen, or in his words and the words of Hippocrates, because the words of
both are mixed in Galen's commentaries to Hippocrates' books; in the case
of others, the sense expressed in the aphorism is partly in Galen's words
and partly in my own; in the case of yet other aphorisms, my own words
express the idea that Galen mentioned. What has prompted me to do so
is the fact that the idea of that aphorism becomes clear only after reading
from scattered places in Galen's lengthy exposition. I have gathered the sum
of the idea of that aphorism and have articulated it in a concise expression.
Since I know that there are more people who blindly follow the opinion of
someone else than people who investigate for themselves and that there are
more deficient people than learned people, I considered it appropriate to
refer, at the end of every aphorism I cite, to that section in Galen's exposition

5   Maimonides, *Medical Aphorisms Treatises 1–5*, edited and translated by Gerrit Bos (Brigham Young
    UP, 2004), 2–3, 61–65, 69. I have removed the editorial bracketing supplied by Bos.

in which he has explained that aphorism. So, if someone has doubts about the wording of that aphorism or about the idea expressed in it, he can easily look up that section and find that aphorism—whether he finds it in Galen's very words, or mostly so, or whether he finds that idea without omission or addition in Galen's exposition in that section, even if it is expressed in different words—so that his doubts are dispelled....

In the name of God, the Merciful, the Compassionate

O Lord, make our task easy

The Fourth Treatise

Containing aphorisms concerning the pulse and the prognostic signs to be derived from it

(1) The existence of the pulse is vital and useful for two things. One of these, the most important, is the maintenance of the innate heat. The second is the generation of the pneuma. *De pulsu* 13.

(2) The meaning of the concept of rhythm mentioned in the different types of the pulse is the ratio of the time of expansion of the arteries to the time of rest which follows, and also of the time of contraction of the arteries to the time of rest which follows. The proportion between these two times is without any doubt according to what is natural for each of the different ages of man. Sometimes it is according to its nature, and sometimes it is different. *De pulsu magna* 1.

(3) Knowledge about the rhythm can be obtained through the strongest possible pulse only. In other types of pulse, the rhythm either cannot be grasped at all or is grasped far from correctly. *De pulsu* 7.

(4) A constant, truthful indicator of the strength of the animal faculty is a strong, equal pulse, and similarly, a great pulse. *De curandi ratione per venae sectionem.*

(5) The pulse of a newborn child is extremely rapid and frequent, while the pulse of old people is extremely slow and rare. The pulses normal for other ages fall between these two by gradation. In the prime of adolescence, the pulse is greatest and strongest. Its greatness and strength diminish gradually until, in old age, it is weakest and smallest. From the time of birth until the prime of adolescence, the pulse gradually increases in greatness and strength. *De pulsu* 11.

...

(11) The first and lowest degree of weakness of the faulty makes the pulse smaller and fainer. The next degree of weakness is that in which one's fingers put on the artery are a burden for the faculty. It turns one's pulse into the recurrent one called "mouse tail." When the faculty is wasted and dissolved even more than this, it turns one's pulse into the permanent "mouse tail." *De pulsu* 10.

...

(18) Sometimes the temperament of the heart is warmer than is necessary and the temperament of the arteries colder than is necessary, or the reverse. Similarly, the body of the heart itself is sometimes cooler than its natural temperament, while the substance contained in the two ventricles of the heart is warmer; or the reverse may occur, in which case the pulse is similar to the natural pulse. These kinds of illnesses lead astray even skilled physicians—let alone other physicians—and cause them to commit mistakes. *De pulsu* 15.

(19) A bad humor often collects in the **cardia** of the stomach and burns it or cools it, so that the pulse becomes small and unequal. The difference between burning and cooling is that the pulse becomes smaller as a result of cooling and it becomes more unequal as a result of burning. *De differentiis febrium* 1.

> **cardia:** The upper opening of the stomach where the esophagus enters.

(20) When biting, pain, pressure, vomiting, fainting, or hiccups occur at the cardia of the stomach, the pulse becomes very spasmodic, small, and weak, and sometimes also rapid. When the cardia of the stomach is compressed or squeezed by a large amount of food or by nonbiting humors streaming to it, the pulse becomes rare, slow, small, and weak. *De pulsu parva.*

(21) If a varying bad temperament occurs in an artery, that part of it containing more moisture and heat has a pulse that is greater and more rapid, whereas the part which is either cold or dry has a pulse that is smaller and slower. *De pulsu* 10.

(22) In the beginning of all the putrefying fevers, the contraction of the artery is more rapid. This is a very reliable diagnostic sign. One should rely on it as a prognostic sign more than on any other sign. A similar thing happens to the pulse when the attacks of these fevers are increasing and intensifying. And, when they reach the state of their culmination, the movements of contraction and expansion of the pulse are less rapid. *De pulsu* 15.

...

(39) The **vermicular** pulse is caused by weakness of the faculty. The undulatory pulse is caused by an excess of moisture and sometimes by extreme softness of the organ. *De pulsu* 10.

> **vermicular:** Worm-like.

DOCUMENT 56:

Al-Rāzī, Case Studies in the Spirit of Hippocrates[6]

Abū Bakr Muhammad ibn Zakariyya al-Rāzī (ca. 865–925 CE), "Rhazes" in Europe, was a physician from Tehran, working in Baghdad, and trained in Arabic-Galenic medicine. Al-Rāzī wrote numerous books on medicine and pharmacy, including a collection of case studies, which seem to come from al-Rāzī's notebook of patient observations and have been loosely arranged into a single treatise. He compares his case studies explicitly to the Hippocratic *Epidemics* (Document 12, pp. 46–48). This is a valuable account of medieval Islamicate medicine in action, as al-Rāzī records his diagnosis, prognosis, treatments, and other clinical observations.

❦

In the name of Allah, the Merciful, the Compassionate!

Illustrative accounts of patients and our own clinical histories, only a mixed record of unusual cases which find their place here on account of their relation to questions and narratives in [Hippocrates'] *Epidemics*. We do not want to delay or postpone this any longer because it is a very useful discussion, particularly on account of the questions raised in it. We had neglected these examples because we intended to collect them all together here. According to this, our intention, we must place the *Epidemics* beside these questions, read them side by side, and write them down here as completely as possible—if Allah will!

[*Case X: Abnormally concentrated urine after a fever.*] Al-'Ibadi suffered from a hot fever. This passed, but the urine remained discolored during many days. His condition improved at times and grew worse again, but his urine showed no difference in its coloration, although the fever went and came again. Thereupon, I made him a venesection, bled him from the **basilic vein** and extracted the blood with the lancet. On the same day his urine became light-colored, and he was completely cured.

[*Case XI: A Case of Smallpox.*] The daughter of al-Husain ibn 'Abdawaih had drunk camel's milk as usual, without asking my advice. When she became **meteoric** after the milk, she took the musk-remedy without having previously submitted herself to a venesection or to purgation. She developed a continuous fever, and there appeared on her body the symptoms

basilic vein: One of the most important veins in premodern bloodletting, traveling on the surface of the inner arm from the shoulder down to the wrist.

meteoric: Suffering from meteorism, a painful swelling of the abdomen or intestines from accumulated gas.

---

6   Max Meyerhof, "Thirty-Three Clinical Observations by Rhazes (Circa 900 A.D.)," *Isis* 23:2 (1935), 321–72: 332, 338–40.

of smallpox; she had, in fact, four attacks of smallpox one after another. When the smallpox began and she consulted me, I took care of her eyes, and strengthened them with **antimony**-powder rubbed in rose-water, and nothing appeared in her eye, although its surroundings were very severely affected. All the people who were near her, wondered at this astonishing fact that her eye was saved. I applied to her for some time barley-water and the like, and her nature did not show any change as is so frequent a consequence of this disorder. There remained some residue of hot fever, and I supposed that this might be because the remainder of the (ill-natured) humors had not been expelled by the usual purgation; I could not venture to obtain an evacuation at once because of the weakening of her forces. So I confined myself to administering to her dried apricots at day-break and barley-water at noon during a fortnight. This procured her two evacuations a day, and she was completely cleared of the disease. The **maturation of the urine** appeared after forty days, and her recovery was complete at the end of fifty days.

[*Case XII: Obesity and Gout.*] Concerning the son of al-Husain ibn Abdawaih, the doctors supposed that he was of a humid temperament on account of his obesity, because they were unable to distinguish between a fleshy man and a fat man. He had an attack of pain in his articulations, which subsided later on. I applied to him several venesections and administered to him once a week containing a remedy which evacuates the yellow bile, because this **nocive** mixture of humors was an acrid purulent matter. I prescribed to him as diet sour, bitter and astringent aliments and forbade him sweets, strong and fatty foods. This disease subsided and caused him only unimportant attacks. When he had followed this prescription for a long time, he was completely restored and his body began simultaneously to lose flesh.

[*Case XIII: Semitertian Fever.*] Ibn Idris was suspected of being attacked by the worst form of **semitertian fever**, the acuteness of which was great; it became chronic while the doctor administered to him pastilles of bamboo-sugar. I prescribed to him to drink barley-water after a dose of **oxymel** and to delay his meal every day until the time of the decrease of the fever and to avoid as much as possible the time of the feverish attack. I insisted upon this prescription, but he found it difficult. I told him, however, "You cannot have any other prescription than this!" Thereupon he followed my advice during several days in my absence, and he came to see me after ten days and was completely restored.

[*Case XIV: A Lacrymal Fistula.*] The son of 'Abd al-Mu'min, the goldsmith, had a lacrymal fistula. I prescribed to him to rub in an eye-wash which I had prepared for him and to insert it by drops into the inner corner; he did this and was healed. I know, however, that this is not a real healing, only a shrinking and drying up of the fistula, but not a clogging; I have experienced that repeatedly. **Galen speaks** of the same matter among his rare cases; it was this that caused me to compound the eye-wash in question.

DOCUMENT 57:

Usamah ibn Munqidh: A Muslim View of Frankish Medicine[7]

Usamah ibn Munqidh (1095–1188 CE) lived in Syria during the era of the Crusades. In this excerpt from his *Memoirs* he describes the medical practices of "Frankish" (Western European Christian) doctors in the Crusader states. Usamah was not a physician himself, but he was a keen observer of human behavior and provides valuable comparisons between European and Islamicate medicine in the twelfth century. He is appalled by some of the Frankish medical techniques, which fail miserably, but is impressed by some of their remedies.

ೕ

The Curious Medication [of the Franks]

A case illustrating their curious medicine is the following: The lord of al-**Munaytirah** wrote to my uncle asking him to dispatch a physician to treat certain sick persons among his people. My uncle sent him a Christian physician named **Thabit**. Thabit was absent but ten days when be returned. So we said to him, "How quickly has thou healed thy patients!" He said:

They brought before me a knight in whose leg an abscess had grown; and a woman afflicted with imbecility. To the knight I applied a small poultice until the abscess opened and became well; and the woman I put on diet and made her humor wet. Then a Frankish physician came to them and said, "This man knows nothing about treating them." He then said to the knight, "Which wouldst thou prefer, living with one leg or dying with two?" The latter replied, "Living with one leg." The physician said, "Bring me a strong knight and a sharp ax." A knight came with the ax. And I was standing by. Then the physician laid the leg of the patient on a block of wood and bade the knight strike his leg with the ax and chop it off at one blow. Accordingly he struck it—while I was looking on—one blow, but the leg was not severed. He dealt another blow, upon which the marrow of the leg flowed out and the patient died on the spot.

He then examined the woman and said, "This is a woman in whose head there is a devil which has possessed her. Shave off her hair." Accordingly they shaved it off and the woman began once more to eat their ordinary diet—garlic and mustard. Her imbecility took a turn for the worse. The physician then said, "The devil has penetrated through her head." He therefore took a

Munaytirah: This was a Crusader fortress in Lebanon, known to the Franks as *Moinestre*.

Thabit: This physician is a Christian, but not a Frank. He has an Arabic name, and it is implied that he practices a superior form of "Arabic" medicine, to be compared to the barbaric "Frankish" medicine.

---

7 *An Arab-Syrian Gentleman and Warrior in the Period of the Crusades: Memoirs of Usamah ibn-Munqidh (Kitab al-i'tibar)*, translated by Philip Hitti (Cornell UP, 1929), 161–62.

razor, made a deep cruciform incision on it, peeled off the skin at the middle of the incision until the bone of the skull was exposed and rubbed it with salt. The woman also expired instantly. Thereupon I asked them whether my services were needed any longer, and when they replied in the negative I returned home, having learned of their medicine what I knew not before.

I have, however, witnessed a case of their medicine which was quite different from that. The king of the Franks had for treasurer a knight named Bernard, who (may Allah's curse be upon him!) was one of the most accursed and wicked among the Franks. A horse kicked him in the leg, which was subsequently infected and which opened in fourteen different places. Every time one of these cuts would close in one place, another would open in another place. All this happened while I was praying for his perdition. Then came to him a Frankish physician and removed from the leg all the ointments which were on it and began to wash it with very strong vinegar. By this treatment all the cuts were healed and the man became well again. He was up again like a devil.

Another case illustrating their curious medicine is the following: In Shayzar we had an artisan named Abu-al-Fath, who had a boy whose neck was afflicted with **scrofula**. Every time a part of it would close, another part would open. This man happened to go to Antioch on business of his, accompanied by his son. A Frank noticed the boy and asked his father about him. Abu-al-Fath replied, "This is my son." The Frank said to him, "Wilt thou swear by thy religion that if I prescribe to you a medicine which will cure thy boy, thou wilt charge nobody fees for prescribing it thyself? In that case, I shall prescribe to you a medicine which will cure the boy." The man took the oath and the Frank said: "Take uncrushed leaves of glasswort, burn them, then soak the ashes in olive oil and sharp vinegar. Treat the scrofula with them until the spot on which it is growing is eaten up. Then take burnt lead, soak it in ghee butter and treat him with it. That will cure him."

The father treated the boy accordingly, and the boy was cured. The sores closed and the boy returned to his normal condition of health. I have myself treated with this medicine many who were afflicted with such disease, and the treatment was successful in removing the cause of the complaint.

scrofula: Painful swelling of the lymph nodes, usually on the neck, and usually caused by tuberculosis.

DOCUMENT 58:

Al-Rāzī on Diagnosis and Treatment for Smallpox and Measles[8]

We met al-Rāzī above in Document 56, imitating the case studies of the
Hippocratic *Epidemics*. Some of his works, like *Kitab al-Jadari wa-al-
Hasba*, or "Book on Smallpox and Measles," display more originality
and a willingness to break with the past. This is one of the first works to
demonstrate differential diagnosis to identify and distinguish between diseases
in a patient. Smallpox and measles present similarly, but al-Rāzī built up a
body of evidence through detailed clinical examinations to distinguish the
one disease from the other. The "Book on Smallpox and Measles" is organized
into 14 chapters, reviewing what the ancients said, detailing the theory of the
disease, and devoting most of the work to practical treatments. In the first
chapter he outlines the causes of smallpox and demonstrates what Galen said
about it and what he did not. This is followed by two chapters on the sorts
of people who are most likely to get smallpox, and in what season, which is
clearly dependent on the Hippocratic work *Airs, Waters, Places* (Document 11,
pp. 42–45), and then an outline of the symptoms of both smallpox and
measles, with advice on how to distinguish the two. The remaining chapters
cover aspects of the prevention and treatment of smallpox and measles, along
with tips for the daily care and diet for those suffering from these diseases.

ev

Chapter 1

*Of the causes of the Small-Pox; how it comes to pass that hardly any one escapes
the disease; and the sum of what Galen says concerning it.*

As to any physician who says that the excellent Galen has made no mention of the Small-Pox, and was entirely ignorant of this disease, surely he
must be one of those who have either never read his works at all, or who
have passed over them very cursorily. For Galen describes a plaster in the
first book of his treatise **Kata genos**, and says that it is useful against this
and that disease, "and also against the Small-Pox." Again, in the beginning
of the fourteenth book of his treatise *On Pulses*, at about the first leaf, he
says, that "the blood is sometimes putrefied in an extraordinary degree, and
that the excess of inflammation runs so high that the skin is burned, and
there break out in it the *Small-Pox* and excoriating erysipelas by which it is

Kata genos: The Greek
means "according to type."
This treatise by Galen
is usually known by its
Latin title *De compositione
medicamentorum
secundum genera* ("On the
composition of medicines
according to type"). It
was translated by Hunayn
ibn Ishaq into Arabic (see
Document 52, p. 153).

---

8   *A Treatise on the Small-Pox and Measles, by Abú Mecr Mohammed ibn Zacaríyá ar-Rází*, translated by
    William Alexander Greenhill (Sydenham Society, 1848). Puncuation modified.

eroded." Again, in the ninth book of his treatise *On the Use of the Members*, he says that "the superfluous parts of the food that remain, which are not converted into blood, and remain in the members, putrefy, and become more acid, in process of time, until there are generated the erysipelas, *Small-Pox*, and spreading inflammation." Again, in the fourth book of ***Timaeus*** he says that "the ancients applied the name *phlegmoun* to everything in which there was inflammation, as the erysipelas, and *Small-Pox*, and that these diseases were in their opinion generated from bile."

If, however, any one says that Galen has not mentioned any peculiar and satisfactory mode of treatment for this disease, nor any complete cause, he is certainly correct; for, unless he has done so in some of his works which have not been published in Arabic, he has made no further mention of it than what we have just cited. As for my own part, I have most carefully inquired of those who use both the Syriac and Greek languages, and have asked them about this matter; but there was not one of them who could add anything to what I have mentioned; and indeed most of them did not know what he meant by those passages which I have distinctly quoted. This I was much surprised at, and also how it was that Galen passed over this disease which occurs so frequently and requires such careful treatment, when he is so eager in finding out the causes and treatment of other maladies.

As to the modern, although they have certainly made some mention of the treatment of the Small-Pox (but without much accuracy and distinctness), yet there is not one of them who has mentioned the cause of the existence of the disease, and how it comes to pass that hardly any one escapes it, or who has disposed the modes of treatment in their right places. And for this reason we hope that the reward of that man who encouraged us to compose this treatise, and also our own, will be doubled, since we have mentioned whatever is necessary for the treatment of this disease, and have arranged and carefully disposed every thing in its right place, by GOD's permission.

We will now begin therefore by mentioning the efficient cause of this distemper, and why hardly any one escapes it; and then we will treat of the other things that relate to it, section by section: and we will (with GOD's assistance) speak on every one of these points with what we consider to be sufficient copiousness.

I say then that every man, from the time of his birth till he arrives at old age, is continually tending to dryness; and for this reason the blood of children and infants is much moister than the blood of young men, and still more so than that of old men. And besides this it is much hotter; as Galen testifies in his Commentary on the *Aphorisms*, in which he says that "the heat of children is greater in quantity than the heat of young men, and the heat of young men is more intense in quality." And this also is evident from

Timaeus: Galen's commentary on Plato's *Timaeus*, which survives only in Arabic, not Greek. See Document 8, pp. 33–34, for a medical passage from the *Timaeus*.

the force with which the natural processes, such as digestion and growth of body, are carried on in children. For this reason the blood of infants and children may be compared to **must**, in which the coction leading to perfect ripeness has not yet begun, nor the movement towards fermentation taken place; the blood of young men may be compared to must, which has already fermented and made a hissing noise, and has thrown out abundant vapors and its superfluous parts, like wine which is now still and quiet and arrived at its full strength; and as to the blood of old men, it may be compared to wine which has now lost its strength and is beginning to grow vapid and sour.

Now the Small-Pox arises when the blood putrefies and ferments, so that the superfluous vapors are thrown out of it, and it is changed from the blood of infants, which is like must, into the blood of young men, which is like wine perfectly ripened: and the Small-Pox itself may be compared to the fermentation and the hissing noise which take place in must at that time. And this is the reason why children, especially males, rarely escape being seized with this disease, because it is impossible to prevent the blood's changing from this state into its second state, just as it is impossible to prevent must (whose nature it is to make a hissing noise and to ferment) from changing into the state which happens to it after its making a hissing noise and its fermentation. And the temperament of an infant or child is seldom such that it is possible for its blood to be changed from the first into the second by little and little, and orderly, and slowly, so that this fermentation and hissing noise should not show itself in the blood: for a temperament, to change thus gradually, should be cold and dry; whereas that of children is just the contrary, as is also their diet, seeing that the food of infants consists of milk; and as for children, although their food does not consist of milk, yet it is nearer to it than is that of other ages; there is also a greater mixture in their food, and more movement after it; for which reason it is seldom that a child escapes this disease. Then afterwards alterations take place in their condition according to their temperaments, regimen, and natural disposition, the air that surrounds them, and the state of the vascular system both as to quantity and quality, for in some individuals the blood flows quickly, in others slowly, in some it is abundant, in other deficient, in some it is very bad in quality, in others less deteriorated...

must: Freshly pressed grape juice and pulp, the first step in winemaking.

Chapter II

A specification of those habits of body which are most disposed to the Small-Pox; and of the seasons in which these habits of body mostly abound.

The bodies most disposed to the Small-Pox are in general such as are moist, pale, and fleshy; the well-colored also, and ruddy, as likewise the swarthy when they are loaded with flesh; those who are frequently attacked by acute and continued fevers, bleeding at the nose, inflammation of the eyes, and white and red pustules, and vesicles; those that are very fond of sweet things, especially dates, honey, figs, and grapes, and all those kinds of sweets in which there is a thick and dense substance, as thick gruel, and honey-cakes, or a great quantity of wine and milk.

Bodies that are lean, bilious, hot, and dry, are more disposed to the Measles than to the Small-Pox; and if they are seized with the Small-Pox, the pustules are necessarily either few in number, distinct, and favorable, or, on the contrary, very bad, numerous, sterile, and dry, with putrefaction, and no maturation....

Chapter III

On the symptoms which indicate the approaching eruption of the Small-Pox and Measles.

The eruption of the Small-Pox is preceded by a continued fever, pain in the back, itching in the nose, and terrors in sleep. These are the more peculiar symptoms of its approach, especially a pain in the back, with fever; then also a pricking which the patient feels all over his body; a fullness of the face, which at times goes and comes; an inflamed color, and vehement redness in both cheeks; a redness of both the eyes; a heaviness of the whole body; great uneasiness, the symptoms of which are stretching and yawning, a pain in the throat and chest, with a slight difficulty in breathing, and cough; a dryness of the mouth, thick spittle, and hoarseness of the voice; pain and heaviness of the head; inquietude, distress of mind, nausea, and anxiety; (with this difference, that the inquietude, nausea, and anxiety are more frequent in the Measles than in the Small-Pox; while, on the other hand, the pain in the back is more peculiar to the Small-Pox than to the Measles;) heat of the whole body, an inflamed color, and shining redness, and especially an intense redness of the gums.

When, therefore, you see these symptoms, or some of the worst of them (such as the pain of the back, and the terrors in sleep, with the continued fever), then you may be assured that the eruption of one or other of these diseases in the patient is nigh at hand....

DOCUMENT 59:

Pilgrim Medicine: Qustā ibn Lūqā on "The Little Dragon of Medina"[9]

The Syrian Christian physician and scientist, Qustā ibn Lūqā (820–912 CE), compiled a health guide for Muslim pilgrims making the *hajj* in his *Medical Regime for the Pilgrims at Mecca*. It is a short treatise of 14 chapters. In the first 12 chapters, Qustā describes topics such as the best times for rest, food, or sexual activity, what winds to avoid, treatments for earaches, the dangers of dust, how to identify healthy water, and so on. The final two chapters (below) concern the treatments for infection from a dangerous parasite, the guinea worm, known then as "the little dragon of Medina" (the city where Muhammad founded Islam). This is still its Latin scientific name: *Dracunculus medinensis*. Qustā outlines medieval theories, shared by all cultures around the Mediterranean, about the spontaneous generation of worms and other small creatures like the guinea worm, ideas which go back to Aristotle.

ۏ

Chapter 13

On the origin of the dracunculus medinensis *and on the prophylaxis against its occurrence.*

Since the *dracunculus medinensis* so often originates in that place, I mean al-Madīna, so that it is known as *medinensis*, I thought it a good thing to describe the regimen which must be the prophylaxis against it. What I want to say is that this worm originates in the flesh in the same way as worms, tapeworms and other kinds of worms originate in the belly, and everything that crawls upon the earth. For all of them occur by way of a common cause: the balanced putrefaction. As putrefaction in the different kinds of matter causes animals, so putrefaction in the flesh causes this worm. Every putrefaction is caused by the combination of heat and moisture in certain quantities. No mortal being, however, can grasp these quantities and no one can know their measures, except the Creator, to Whom belong glory and greatness. For these quantities are not subject to limitation, neither increase nor decrease adheres to them.

They are, however, liable to difference and this difference is analogous to that of the animals which originate from them. For the quantities of heat and moisture from which worms in the belly originate differ from

---

9 Gerrit Bos, translator, *Qusta Ibn Luqa's Medical Regime for the Pilgrims to Mecca. The Risala fi tadbir safar al-hajj* (Leiden, 1992), 73–81. Punctuation modified.

those from which tapeworms originate and from those from which ticks, fleas, gnats and bugs originate. Just as the quantities from which lizards, jerboas and rats are born from the earth differ from the quantities from which snakes, scorpions and cockroaches are born. And differing animals are born in different countries analogous to the different kinds of soil of those countries. For every country is distinguished by its own kind of soil, from which animals are born which are different from those born in another kind of soil. The animals born in fertile soil, for instance, are different from those born in ashy soil, and the animals born in red soil differ from those born in black soil. If there is putrefaction in one kind of soil, its measures are different from those from which animals are born in another kind of soil. The species of animals born in one country are therefore so different from the species born in another country that in some countries the species of scorpion, in other countries that of fleas and in still other countries that of bugs, does not occur.

In this way the *dracunculus medinensis* is mostly born in al-Madīna, but not in other places. The reason for this is that the climate of that place and the kinds of food with which people feed themselves, such as dates, cause this worm to appear in the flesh and to become an animal like the other animals born in the stomach and intestines. One can protect oneself against its occurrence by: 1) totally giving up the eating of dates. 2) being careful not to use those kinds of food which deteriorate quickly, such as the different kinds of milk and the products made of it, such as cheese, whey and the like. 3) taking a warm bath frequently or pouring warm water over one's body in that country where one cannot take a warm bath. 4) drinking much oxymel before taking food. 5) taking the electuary of yellow **myrobolan** in the daytime; the confection of chebulic myrobolan, of emblic myrobolan and of **secacul**. 6) taking pills which clean the stomach and intestines, such as the pill known as *shaybār*, the pill of gold and the pill of bdellium. 7) taking the powder of chebulic myrobolan, fennel, sugar and the like. 8) using the caper plant for a decoction.

Preparing **collyria** from the stalk and fruit of the caper plant is one of the most useful remedies against this disease. The same applies to dill, fennel, dandelion, water mint, mountain mint, rue, peppermint and all the vegetables. They open the pores of the body, boil its humors and bring them into a state of balance so they neither get stuck nor cause putrefaction in any member of the body. By this regimen and what resembles it one can protect oneself against the *dracunculus medinensis*, God willing.

myrobolan: Myrobolans are a small type of plum from the Middle East and South Asia, but which have now spread through Eurasia. They were a popular ingredient in Near Eastern medicines and spread to Europe during the eleventh century.

secacul: A member of the carrot and celery family (*Apiaceae*) used in medieval Islamicate medicine, either the skirret (*Sium sisarum*) or a type of parsnip (*Malabaila secacul*).

collyria: Collyrium (singular), eye salves.

Chapter 14

On the description of the treatment of the dracunculus medinensis *once it has appeared in the stomach.*

It is good and praiseworthy to have some knowledge of what is useful against it, even if there is no urgent need for it. I therefore thought it a good thing to give this description of the treatment of the *dracunculus medinensis*, even if Hippocrates and Galen do not mention it. I want to quote the opinion of Soranus and Leonidas, two exemplary physicians. Soranus thought that this worm is not an animal and that it does not move; it only seems to move, but does not move in reality. Leonidas and other physicians after him thought that it is an animal which originates in the flesh of the muscles, mostly in the forearms and upper arms, in the legs and thighs. As for boys it also originates in the back and chest under the skin.

All these physicians agree concerning its treatment that one should constantly foment the limb in which the worm appears with warm water until its end comes out. And when it comes out one should softly pull it. But if it does not want to come out completely, one should tie a piece of lead with a thread to its end. Then one should leave it alone so the piece of lead can pull it out by its weight little by little. Besides one should make the patient sit in warm water and bind the area affected with dissolving dressings such as the one prepared from the flour of barley, flour of wheat, fenugreek, figs, chamomile and the like. One should also stick dissolving plasters on the wound, such as the one named after the laurel, the tamarisk and other, similar ones. If, however, the *dracunculus medinensis* breaks off and the place is open, the rest should be taken out and the wound should be treated as other wounds. I have come to the end of what was necessary to say about the treatment of the *dracunculus medinensis*, for which I used the same method as for the rest of my treatise....

Ancient Greeks in Later Medieval Prophetic Medicine: *'Al-Tibb al-Nabawī*[10]

Al-Suyūtī (ca. 1445–1505 CE), also known as Jalaluddin, was an Egyptian religious scholar and prolific author of commentaries on the Quran. One of his works, *'Al-Tibb al-Nabawī*, synthesizes centuries of scholarship on the "Medicine of the Prophet" (see Document 45, pp. 132–33 on this tradition) and combines it with teachings from Hippocrates, Galen, Avicenna, and other rational physicians.

ev

Said 'Ali ibn al-Hussayn ibn Wafid: God has collected all Medicine into half a verse when He said: Eat and drink but not to excess.

Said 'Umr: Avoid a pot-belly, for it spoils the body, breeds disease, and renders prayer wearisome. Take to blood-letting for this rectifies the body. And avoid all excess. For God hates a learned man who is fat. This is reported by Abu Nu'aim.

Said Hippocrates: The continuation of good health depends upon moderate labour and the avoidance of a surfeit of eating and drinking. He also said: A little of what is harmful is better than a lot of what is good.

Said al-Shahrastani in his book entitled *Al-Milal wa al-Nihal* or *The Book of Religions and Sects*: Hippocrates is the founder of Medicine. And he added: Our ancestors and those who came later prefer him to all. A certain Greek king sent to him several **qantars** of gold and asked him to come and visit him. But he refused. He also used to refuse any fee for treating the poor or men of middle means. But he stipulated that he should take from the rich one of three things—a collar of gold or a diadem or golden bracelets.

When asked what life is the best Hippocrates answered: Safety with poverty is better than wealth with fear. He also said: Every man should be treated with herbals from his own country. When he was dying he said: Recognise one who seeks learning from his much sleep, his mild nature, his soft skin, and his long life.

He also said: Had Man been created with a single constitution, he would never have suffered sickness. For then there would have been nothing in opposition to cause disease.

qantar: Also *kantar*, a large unit of weight in the Eastern Mediterranean, today 45.02 kg in Egypt.

---

10 Al-Suyūtī, *'Al-Tibb al-Nabawī*, translated by Cyril Elgood in "Tibb-ul-Nabi or Medicine of the Prophet," *Osiris* 14 (1962), 33–192: 54–55.

A physician once visited a sick man and said to him: You, the disease and I are three. If by hearkening to me you help me, then we shall be two against one and thus stronger. And when two come against one, they defeat it.

Hippocrates was once asked: Why does a man when he is dead, weigh more than when he was alive? He replied: Once he was made up of two parts, a light part lifting him up and a heavy part weighing him down. When one of these went away, and it was the light part that does the lifting that went, then the heavy part weighs him down yet more.

He once said to one of his students: Let your best means of treating people be your love for them, your interest in their affairs, your knowledge of their condition, and your recognised attentiveness to them.

He also said: All excess is against Nature. Let your food, your drink, your sleep, and your sexual intercourse be all in moderation.

And he said: Any physician who administers a poison or procures an **abortion** or prevents a pregnancy or prolongs the disease of a sick man, this physician is no colleague of mine. On this subject he composed a well-known oath which I shall discuss later, if God wills.

The books by Hippocrates on Medicine are many. Among them are the *Book of Aphorisms*, the *Book of Prognostics*, and the **Kitab Qubra Buqrat**. This last book testifies to many wonders of wonders. When the tombs of several of the Greek kings were opened, this book was found inside.

abortion: In premodern and early modern texts, the term was used both for intentional abortion of the fetus and unintentional miscarriages. But here, as in the oaths of Hippocrates and Asaph above, intentional abortion is clearly meant.

Book of Aphorisms: See Document 10, pp. 39–41, for selections from the *Aphorisms*, which became central to medical education in both European and Islamicate cultures.

Book of Prognostics: Another of the most famous Hippocratic works, quite possibly by the real Hippocrates, which provided instructions for making a prognosis of a disease based on the observation of the patient's symptoms. It became, along with the *Aphorisms*, one of the fundamental works of medieval medical education.

Kitab Qubra Buqrat: This last work Is not part of the usual Hippocratic Corpus. Its description is similar to the Pseudo-Hippocratic work known in Latin as *Capsula Eburnea* (*The Ivory Casket*). According to the standard version of that work, however, it was found in the tomb of Hippocrates himself and not of Greek kings.

PART 8

Learned Medicine in High Medieval Europe (ca. 1000–1400 CE)

HUMORS, COMPLEXION, AND UROSCOPY (DOCUMENTS 61–65)

The documents and images in this chapter come from Latin Europe during the central and high Middle Ages (ca. 1000–1400 CE), a period which saw European physicians rediscover ancient Greek medicine either through Late Antique Latin works or through Arabic medical books like those in Part 7. Learned physicians and philosophers of high medieval Europe focused on the humoral theory described by Hippocrates, Galen, and their later commentators. Sources 61–65 demonstrate two of the most important aspects of learned medicine in this period: treatment based on the identification of an individual's humoral "complexion" and diagnosis based on the analysis of urine (uroscopy). Even though both Hippocrates and Galen mention urine in their diagnoses and prognoses, it was only in the Middle Ages that formalized uroscopy became a central aspect of medical practice, first in Byzantine Alexandria and then in medieval Islamicate and European cultures.

Learned medicine, with its focus on diagnosis from bodily signs and treatment based on the manipulation of humors, disappeared almost entirely from Western Europe in the fifth through eleventh centuries. Document 61, from the tenth century in German lands, is thus rare in reflecting some of this learned tradition. The author, Ekkehard IV (ca. 980–1056), was a monk at the wealthy abbey of St. Gall (now in Switzerland). In his chronicle of the abbey, Ekkehard describes a humorous episode in which the monk Notker II "the Physician" (d. 975) tricks Duke Henry of Bavaria using his knowledge of uroscopy.

About a century after Notker II lived Constantine the African (Constantinus Africanus, d. ca. 1098), a North African Christian who became a monk at the famous Abbey of Montecassino in Italy, founded by St. Benedict (see Document 43, pp. 128–29). Montecassino was not only a famous religious center but also an important location for learning and translation in the central Middle Ages (ca. 900–1100 CE). Constantine, probably a native speaker of Arabic, translated or adapted around 20 medical works from Arabic into Latin, including the *Isagoge* of Johannitius (Document 52, pp. 153–57). One of his largest and most ambitious projects was a translation and adaptation of the *Complete Book of the Medical Art* by the tenth-century Persian-Arabic physician 'Ali ibn al-'Abbas al-Majusi, known in Latin as Haly Abbas. Constantine named his work the *Pantegni* (Document 62), from the Greek *pan-techne*, or "whole art," and it usually circulated as his own composition.[1] The *Pantegni* quickly became one of the core texts of scholarly medical education first in southern Italy and then throughout all of Latin Europe during the twelfth century.

European medicine was transformed during the "long twelfth century" (ca. 1075–1225) by the translation of Arabic medical works like the *Isagoge* and *Pantegni* as well as long-lost Greek works by or attributed to Hippocrates and Galen. The new European medicine is often called "Salernitan" after the southern Italian port city of Salerno, which was renowned for its learned physicians. The location of Salerno in the middle of the Mediterranean Sea opened it to significant contacts from North African and Near Eastern cultures, which included both peaceful trading and violent raiding. One of the intercultural benefits of Salerno was a vibrant medical culture that benefited from the presence of Latin and Greek Christians, Muslims, and Jews. Salerno also had close connections with the nearby city of Naples and the abbey of Montecassino, home of Constantine the African and other scholars.

By the turn of the twelfth century "Salerno" became almost a brand name for learned (and often expensive) medicine practiced by scholarly physicians trained in the physiology and therapeutics of Hippocrates, Galen, and Avicenna (Documents 53 and 54, pp. 158–64). Physicians and wise women come from Salerno in several works of high medieval literature.[2] The later twelfth-century theologian Peter the Chanter paints the portrait of a sinner who cares more for this world than the next: he "cares more for his body than his soul, running to Salerno, consulting the physicians, studying civil law, neglecting divine law, spending more on his body and the world than

---

1   The oldest surviving copy of the *Pantegni*, prepared perhaps under the direction of Constantine himself at the abbey of Montecassino, is fully digitized and described online: www.kb.nl/en/themes/medieval-manuscripts/liber-pantegni.

2   See Stephanie Cain Van d'Elden, "The Salerno Effect: The Image of Salerno in Courtly Literature," in *L'imaginaire courtois et son double*, edited by Giovanna Angeli and Luciano Formisano, Pubblicazioni dell' Università degli Studi di Salerno, Sezione Atti, Convegni, Miscellanee 35 (Naples, 1992), 503–15.

on his soul and heaven."[3] For Peter, writing in Paris, Salerno had become synonymous with learned, natural, and expensive medicine.

So-called Salernitan doctors did not need to be in or from Salerno itself. For that reason, we do not know who wrote the *Regimen Sanitatis Salernitanum* (Document 63), "The Regimen of Health from Salerno," a Latin poem from the twelfth century outlining the basics of a rationalized diet and physiology associated with Salernitan physicians. The *Regimen* was immensely popular and was expanded by many authors during the later Middle Ages. Different versions survive in manuscript, ranging widely from about 1,000 to 5,000 lines of verse.

The medieval science of uroscopy grew increasingly complicated, as European physicians built on the older Byzantine and Arabic traditions of reading urine for diagnosis and prognosis. Document 64 reproduces a fourteenth-century "urine wheel," a diagram showing twenty different colors of urine and their medical significance. The manuscript illumination in Document 65 presents an idealized vision of how a medieval physician engaged in uroscopy. This physician, however, is none other than Constantine the African, whose name and image lend greater authority to the art of uroscopy.

---

3 Peter the Chanter, *Summa de sacramentis et animae consiliis* II, cap. 112, edited by Jean-Albert Dugauquier, 6 vols. (Éditions Nauwelaerts, 1954).

DOCUMENT 61:

A Clever Duke and a Cleverer Physician in Tenth-Century Europe[4]

Ekkehard IV (ca. 980–1056) was a monk and historian at the wealthy abbey of St. Gall, where he wrote the *Casus Sancti Galli*, a historical chronicle of his monastery. In this work, Ekkehard describes the humorous meeting of Notker II "the Physician" (d. 975), a monk at St. Gall, with Duke Henry of Bavaria. Notker's skill as a physician is attributed to his knowledge of Hippocrates' *Aphorisms* (Document 10, pp. 39–41) and *Prognostics*. Hippocratic medicine taught him how to make medical diagnoses and prognoses from urine (uroscopy) and he uses this knowledge to turn the tables on the Duke when he tried to trick him.

℘

Let us speak briefly, before hastening on to other matters, about Notker, a teacher, painter, and doctor, since we have enough material for a large volume. He made many pictures for St. Gall after the fire, as one can see on the doors and ceiling of the church and in certain books. But what are these matters compared to the thousand other things, which made him famous as a teacher and healer? ... As a healer he frequently performed marvellous and stupendous works, because he was uniquely learned in medical *Aphorisms*, spices as well as antidotes, and the *Prognostics* of Hippocrates, as could be seen in the case of the urine of **Duke Henry**, who craftily tried to deceive him. He sent to Notker the urine of a certain young chambermaid for him inspect, and Notker said, "God is about to perform an unheard of miracle and portent, that a man should give birth from his womb. For the Duke himself, about thirty days from today, will lay upon his breast the child brought forth from his womb." The duke, at last caught out, blushed, and sent gifts to this man of God so that he would not refuse to serve as his doctor, for he had been brought there for that purpose. The doctor of St. Gall also brought that young woman, at her request, back into the duke's favor, for just as he had foretold by means of prognosis, she did give birth to a child.

He also quickly soothed a long-standing bloody nose for our Bishop Kaminold (of Konstanz). But, smelling the blood, Notker foretold that a case of smallpox would befall the bishop in three days. When the bishop begged that he stop the pustules erupting on him on the very day that he foretold, Notker replied: "To be sure, I could do that, but I will not, because

Duke Henry: Probably Duke Henry II "the Quarrelsome" of Bavaria (r. 955–76, 985–95).

---

4   *Ekkehardi IV. Casus S. Galli*, edited by von Arx, in *Monumenta Germaniae Historica. Scriptores II: Scriptores rerum Sangallensium. Annales, chronica et historiae aevi Carolini*, edited by G.H. Pertz (Hanover, 1829), 136. Original translation by the editor of this volume.

I could not suffer so many penances for being guilty of your murder. For, if I should try to treat these pustules, I would deliver you to death." But at last he did heal the erupted pustules in so short a time, that there remained no sign of even a single mark.

Constantine the African, *Pantegni*: Understanding Complexion[5]

> Constantine the African (d. ca. 1098), a North African monk at the Abbey
> of Montecassino in Italy, was one of the most important medical scholars
> of the Middle Ages even though he did not practice medicine himself. He
> translated or adapted around 20 Arabic medical works into Latin, including
> the *Isagoge* of Johannitius (Document 52, pp. 153–57) and the *Kitab al-Maliki*,
> or *Complete Book of the Medical Art*, by the tenth-century Persian-Arabic
> physician al-Majusi. Constantine called his translation *Pantegni* (Greek for
> "the whole art") and it usually circulated as his own composition. The *Kitab
> al-Maliki* contained two parts, one on medical theory (*Theorica*) and one on
> medical practice (*Practica*), each containing 10 books. Constantine, however,
> completed only part of his translation (sometime before 1086), finishing
> all of the *Theorica* but only three books of the *Practica*. Later disciples of
> Constantine, seeking a truly complete Latin version, added excerpts from
> other works on practical medicine to complete a 10-book *Practica* to match
> the 10-book *Theorica*. The excerpt below comes from the first book of the
> *Theorica* of the *Pantegni*, in which Constantine outlines the basic medical
> doctrine of "complexion."

e

Chapter 6. On Changes in Complexion

In the above treatise on the elements, we proved that all bodies are subject
to growth and decay from the mixing of the elements in different quantity
and quality according to what is needed for the formation of a true body.
Quantity is either equal or unequal; so let the equal therefore be called
"temperate" and the unequal "intemperate," in which two of the four qualities is in excess. We call that thing "complexion" which is composed from
a mixture of the elements. Therefore if a body composed of the elements
is equal in quantity and quality, it will be "temperate." If the fiery part is in
excess, it is hot; if the airy, it is humid; if the watery, cold; if the earthy, dry;
if the fiery and airy, hot and humid; if airy and watery, cold and humid; if
watery and earthy, cold and dry; if fiery and earthy, hot and dry.

There are therefore nine complexions: eight unequal and one equal. Of
the unequal there are four simple and four composite, and two in the greatest
extremity, for one extremity is temperate, the other intemperate, between

---

5   Constantine the African, *Pantegni, Theorica* I, cap. vi–vii, printed as a work of Isaac Israeli in *Omnia
    Opera Ysaac* (Lyons, 1515). Original translation by the editor of this volume.

which there are many degrees. For example, if we mix different colors, like white and black, yellow and red, in equal weight, we produce colors different from the first. But if we diminish one part, and add the other back, that second color is returned, and so on into infinity. Whence it happens concerning complexions, on account of the diversity of quantities in bodies, that there their forms appear to be different.

Chapter 7. On the Division of Complexions

Many people divide each one of the complexions in various ways: they say one is temperate, the other intemperate. The temperate is equal in the complexions of all its extremities, containing in equal measure a quantity from the mixture of the four elements. That complexion is equal and very true and separated. There is another complexion which is temperate according to what is the necessary temperament of any given body. But human bodies are certainly and truly in the neighborhood of "temperate," and although brute animals are content with only one activity, one and the same human is prepared for all things. He is therefore rational and intellectual, because he understands what he does and discerns with his reason. The hands, for example, are more temperate than the rest of the body, so they can more easily touch touchable things and hold more firmly onto things to be held. For if touch were not temperate, it could not discern hot from cold, nor soft from hard, nor gentle from harsh things. Nobody feels something unless sensation is changed into the quality of the thing sensed. For example, it was proper that the sense of touch in a man was temperate to hold onto things needing to be held. For if hands were excessively soft or hard they could not grip things needing to be gripped, but nevertheless it is fitting that a person holding something be harder rather than soft. Concerning a temperate complexion, Galen spoke thus: No body can be discovered with the senses or intellect to be equally temperate in all extremities. For some body can be conceived in the mind composed equally of four qualities, nevertheless one quality is understood to inhere which is assimilated to none of the other, and this is said to be "temperate."

But if we wish to understand according to our senses, let us mix an equal weight of very hot water and very cold snow. If they are mixed together and touched, they are found to be temperate between hot and cold. If we mix dust and water we feel them to be temperate between soft and hard, and so we can propose many similar things by which "temperate" can be understood, but "temperate" according to what is necessary in every body and in all extremities it is certainly and truthfully temperate and equal according what is necessary for the shape of the body in which it is established. For example, a lion is rather hot, so it is fast and fierce. A rabbit is cold, so it is timid and apt to flee. Every complexion is discerned to be more temperate according to its purpose, just as a horse is called temperate because it is swift and suited for battle, a dog is similarly "temperate" because it is skillful in hunting and familiar with its master's call. The same can be understood in things growing from the earth, for a grape vine and a fig are said to be "temperate" because they are very fruitful and possess a good flavor. Similarly in the case of flavors and spices, those ones are said to be "temperate" which help better according to their own nature. It is sufficient to speak about the temperament of a complexion according to what is necessary....

DOCUMENT 63:

Simplified Humoral Medicine in Verse: The Salernitan Regimen of Health[6]

> The *Regimen Sanitatis Salernitanum* ("The Regimen of Health from Salerno")
> is a lengthy Latin poem from the early twelfth century outlining the basics
> of Salernitan diet and physiology. It may not have been written in Salerno,
> as some versions are dedicated to the king of England. Much of the text
> could easily come from the early Middle Ages, as it is similar to the dietary
> advice of Oribasius and Anthimus (Documents 34 and 35, pp. 104–08). But
> other sections present more contemporary, Salernitan descriptions of the
> four humors and the temperaments expected from a person with a sanguine,
> bilious, phlegmatic, or melancholic complexion.

❧

Salerno's school, in conclave high, unites
To counsel England's King, and thus indites:
If thou to health and vigor wouldst attain,
Shun weighty cares—all anger deem profane,
From heavy suppers and much wine abstain.
Not trivial count it, after pompous fare,
To rise from table and to take the air.
Shun idle, noonday slumber, nor delay
The urgent calls of Nature to obey.
These rules if thou wilt follow to the end,
Thy life to greater length thou mayst extend.
Shouldst doctors need? Be these in Doctors' stead—
Rest, cheerfulness, and table thinly spread....

Let noontide sleep be brief, or none at all;
Else stupor, headache, fever, rheums will fall
On him who yields to noontide's drowsy call....

Four ills from long-imprisoned flatus flow,
Convulsions, colics, dropsies, vertigo;
The truth of this the things itself doth show.

---

6   John Ordronaux, translator, *Regimen Sanitatis Salernitanum. Code of Health of the School of Salernum*
    (J.B. Lippincott & Co., 1871), 47–55, 91–93, 115–19. Slightly modified with reference to Virginia de
    Frutos González, editor and translator, *Flos medicine (Regimen sanitatis Salernitanum)* (Valladolid,
    2012).

Great suppers will the stomach's peace impair.
Wouldst lightly rest? Curtail thine evening fare.
Eat not again till thou dost certain feel
Thy stomach freed of all its previous meal.
This mayst thou know from hunger's teasing call,
Or mouth that waters—surest sign of all! ...

The luscious peach, the apple and the pear,
Cheese, venison, salted meats and even the hare,
With flesh of goats, dyspeptic throes provoke,
And crush the weak beneath melancholy's yoke.
Salt is the flesh of ruffled ducks and geese;
Fried meats do harm; while boiled give peptic peace;
And fragrant roasts, digestive powers increase.
Bitters will purge—crude things in all cause wind,
And salted meats the body dry and bind,
While crusts give rise to bile of darkest kind.
Salt things consume virility and sight,
And **psoric** torments breed of direst might.

psoric: Relating to psoriasis and other painful, inflamed skin conditions.

Eggs newly laid and broths of richest juice,
With ruby wine, increase of strength produce,
Wheat and milk make flesh, brains and tender cheese,
Marrow and pork, as taste they chance to please.
Or eggs with art prepared, or honeyed wine;
Ripe figs and grapes, fresh gathered from the vine....

We hold that men, on no account, should vary
Their daily diet until necessary;
For, as Hippocrates doth truly show,
Diseases sad from all such changes flow.
A stated diet, as it is well known,
Of physic is the strongest corner-stone.
By means of which, if you can naught impart,
Relief of cure, vain is your Healing Art.

Doctors should thus their patient's food revise—
What is it? When the meal? And what its size?
How often? Where? Lest, by some sad mistake,
Ill-sorted things should meet and trouble make....

Four humors form the body in this style,
Atrabilis, blood, phlegm, and yellow bile.
With earth atrabilis may well compare,
Consuming fire with bile, and blood with air.
Blood is moist, warm, and vital as the air;
While phlegm is cold, through water's copious share;
Bile burns like fire, wherever it flows along;
Gall, dry and cool, to earth bears likeness strong.

The Sanguine

Such are by nature stout, and sprightly too,
And ever searching after gossip new.
Love Venus, Bacchus, banquets, noisy joy,
And jovial, they kind words alone employ;
In studies apt—pre-eminent in arts,
No wrath from any cause ever moves their hearts.
Gay, loving, cheerful and profuse in all,
Hearty, tuneful, wherever fate may call;
They're florid, bold, and yet benign withal.

The Bilious Temperament

With headstrong people yellow bile sorts well,
For such men would in everything excel.
They learn with ease—eat much and grow apace,
Are great, profuse, an avid of high place.
Hairy, bold, wrathful, crafty, lavish, shrewd,
Their form is lithe, **complexion** saffron-hued.

The Phlegmatic Temperament

Phlegm breadth imparts, slight power and stature short,
Forms fat, and blood of an inferior sort.
Such men love ease, not books—their bodies steep,
And heavy minds and slothful lives in sleep.
Sluggish and dull their senses almost fail;
They're fat, to spitting prone; their mien is pale.

complexion: In medieval medical texts "complexion" usually refers to the combination of qualities and humors in every person, plant, animal, or food, but here it has the modern sense of the tone and color of one's skin.

The Melancholy Temperament

Of dark Atrabilis we've next to learn—
Which renders man sad, base and taciturn;
In studies keen, in mind not prone to sleep,
In enterprise unfaltering to keep.
Doubting, artful, sad, sordid misers, they
Are timid, while their hue resembles clay.

Behold the diverse humors which bestow
Varied complexions on all here below;
From phlegm a pale complexion comes in all,
A dusky or florid from blood or gall.

DOCUMENT 64:

A Medieval Urine Wheel[7]

The medieval science of uroscopy grew increasingly complicated, as can be seen in Documents 54 (pp. 162–64), 61 (pp. 186–87), and 80 (p. 240). The physician had to analyze the color, smell, texture, separation, and even taste of the patient's urine to help with diagnosis and prognosis. Medical handbooks in the later medieval ages frequently included charts, keyed to accompanying texts, to help the physician determine the urine's color, which could range from more typical "white" and "yellow" to the more obviously dangerous "red" and "black." This fourteenth-century manuscript version is a typical urine wheel, including 20 different colors and their medical significance.

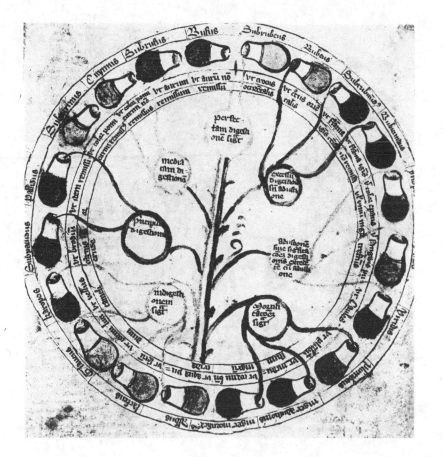

---

7 Universitätsbibliothek Leipzig MS 1177, fol. 28 (fourteenth century).

DOCUMENT 65:

Constantine the African with a Urine Glass[8]

By the later Middle Ages, Constantine the African had become one of the great authorities on medicine, even though he wasn't actually a practicing physician and he translated rather than wrote himself most of the works under his name. In this fourteenth-century manuscript illumination, Constantine is portrayed as a monk, a scholar, and a physician, as men and women come to him with urine glasses for examination. Compare their shape with the urine glasses shown in Document 64. This sort of jar became a popular symbol for medicine in the later Middle Ages, just as a stethoscope can stand today for learned medicine.

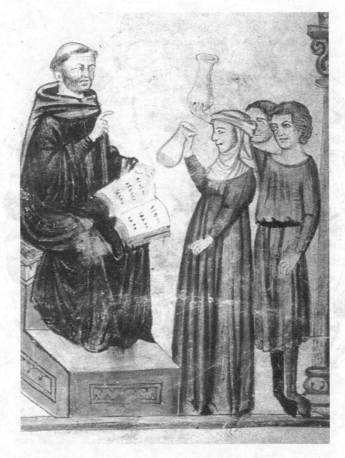

---

8   From a mid-fourteenth-century Italian medical treatise.

EXPLAINING DISEASES (DOCUMENTS 66–68)

One of the concepts in medieval medicine that is most foreign to modern readers is their notion of disease. We have been taught for the last century and more that many diseases are caused by microscopic organisms: pathogenic bacteria and viruses. According to modern bacteriology, specific pathogens cause specific illnesses and to treat the illness you remove or destroy the pathogen. But premodern medicine, without the germ theory developed in the later nineteenth century, considered disease to be mostly a personal matter, caused by the imbalance of one's own humors or as a supernatural punishment for one's own behavior. Diseases were defined by sets of symptoms, and thus as a patient's symptoms changed, the diagnosis and treatment could also change. But even within the medieval Arabic-Galenic system of medical theory, certain diseases were recognized as distinct entities that did not necessarily follow the usual humoral explanations.

Many of the diseases and conditions described by medieval physicians, like smallpox, measles, and Guinea worm disease (see Documents 58 and 59, pp. 173–79), are still recognizable today, even if we treat them differently. But some medieval "diseases" are no longer the concern of physicians, such as *eros*, a crippling form of lovesickness. Constantine the African, and other Late Antique and medieval authors, described this disease, providing learned descriptions of its cause and treatments. In one of his works (Document 66), known as the *Viaticum* ("provision for a journey"), Constantine medicalizes love by explaining its development, benefits, and dangers using rationalized humoral medical theory.

One of the most challenging diseases to diagnose and treat in the Middle Ages was leprosy. *Lepra* (the Greek and Latin term) could apply to a wide range of skin and nerve conditions and not just Hansen's Disease (the preferred name now for leprosy). A representative medieval author on the subject of leprosy is Platearius, an author-physician of the Salernitan school of medicine in the twelfth century, and a direct intellectual descendant of Constantine. He was most likely related to Matthaeus Platearius, the supposed author of the learned herbal *Circa instans* (Document 75, pp. 226–27). Platearius's most popular work was his *Practica* (Document 67), so named because it is dedicated to the practical treatment of specific conditions, and is thus not about *theorica*, or the theoretical explanation of the causes of diseases and of how medicines worked. The work is organized, like most medical treatises of the later Middle Ages, in a head-to-toe fashion. One of its longest passages concerns the identification and treatment of leprosy.

The medieval disease *par excellence* is, of course, bubonic plague, which hit Europe and the Near East in three great waves, or pandemics: the

First Pandemic, or Plague of Justinian, ca. 540–750 (see Documents 46–48, pp. 134–40); the Second Pandemic (ca. 1330–1720); and the Third Pandemic (1859–present day), which is global and still endemic in places such as Madagascar, the Democratic Republic of the Congo, and the southwestern United States. Most people know about bubonic plague from its deadliest strike on the Near East and Europe in 1346–53, the era of the "Black Death." Numerous authors from European, Byzantine, and Islamicate cultures recorded the impact of plague at this time. The French physician Guy de Chauliac (ca. 1300–68) describes the causes, spread, and symptoms of plague in his *Chirurgia Magna*, "Great Surgery" (Document 68), written around 1360. While many contemporary documents survive from the time of the Black Death, few were written by active medical practitioners.

DOCUMENT 66:

Diagnosing Lovesickness: Constantine the African's Medicalized Emotions[9]

Constantine the African and other Late Antique and medieval authors described lovesickness as a disease, providing learned descriptions of its cause and treatments. In this passage from his medical textbook *Viaticum*, Constantine medicalizes love by interpreting its causes, effects, and cures through the lens of Galenic medical theory. He also prescribes poetry and the company of friends as remedies for this disease. This is not simply good psychological advice, but an example of how every substance, action, and emotion was interpreted during the High Middle Ages through a humoral, medical framework.

ℰ

The love called *eros* is a disease related to the brain. It is a great desire with excessive lust and a tormenting of the thoughts, for which reason some philosophers say: *Eros* is a name designating the greatest delight. Just as faithfulness is the perfected form of delight, so also *eros* is a certain extreme form of delight.

Sometimes the excessive need for this sort of love is the need of nature to expel a great superfluity of humors. Concerning this **Rufus** says, "Intercourse seems to benefit those in whom black bile and manic behavior are dominant. Sensation is returned to him and the *erotic* annoyance is removed, if he **interacts** even with those he does not love." Sometimes the cause of *eros* is also the consideration of beautiful shapeliness. If the soul observes this in a form very similar to itself, it goes mad, it seems, for accomplishing the fulfillment of its desire for it.

Since this infirmity may have more dangerous outcomes for the soul, namely, overwrought thought, the eyes of those [with *eros*] always become hollow, always moving quickly on account of the soul's ideas and cares for finding and possessing those things which they desire. Their eyelids are heavy and their skin color becomes yellowish. This happens because of the movement of heat, which is the outcome of their sleepless nights. The pulse hardens, does not dilate naturally, nor is its beat preserved according to what is fitting.

Rufus: Rufus of Ephesus, a Roman writer of the first or second century CE. He wrote a treatise on melancholy, which was known only in fragments during the Middle Ages. See his *Medical Questions* above in Document 21, pp. 74–75.

interacts: The verb translated here, *loquatur*, usually means speaking, but here it is a euphemism for the sexual act.

---

9   Constantine the African, *Viaticum* I.20, in *Lovesickness in the Middle Ages. The* Viaticum *and Its Commentaries*, edited by Mary F. Wack (U of Pennsylvania P, 1990), 186–90. Original translation by the editor of this volume.

If the patient sinks into thoughts, the action of the soul and body is damaged, since the body follows the soul in its action, and the soul accompanies the body in its **passion**. "The power of the soul," Galen says, "follows the complexion of the body." Thus if erotic lovers are not helped so that their thought is lifted and their spirit lightened, they inevitably fall into a melancholic disease. And just as they fall into a troublesome disease from excessive bodily labor, so they also fall into melancholy from labor of the soul.

The following helps erotic lovers better so that they do not sink into excessive thoughts: temperate and fragrant wine is to be given; listening to music; conversing with dearest friends; recitation of poetry; looking at bright, sweet-smelling and fruitful gardens having clear running water; walking or amusing themselves with good looking women or men. "Wine," Rufus says, "is a strong medication for the sad, the timid, and erotic lovers." Galen: "Whoever first strove to press wine from the vines is to be reckoned among the most wise." **Zeno** said: "Just as the bitterness of **lupines** is removed by infusing them in water, so the harshness of my spirit is changed into sweetness after drinking wine." Again, Rufus says: "Not only wine, temperately drunk, relieves sadness, but indeed similar things, like a temperate bath." Thus it happens that when certain people enter a bath they are moved to sing. Therefore certain philosophers say that sound is like the spirit and wine like the body, each of which is aided by the other. Others say that Orpheus said: "Emperors invite me to banquets so that they may take pleasure in me, but I delight equally in them; as I wish I am able to bend their spirits from anger to mildness, from sadness to joy, from avarice to liberality, from fear to boldness." This is the regulation of music and wine for the health of the spirit.

passion: The Latin word *passio* means any kind of suffering, which includes our modern meaning of passion as sexual excitement or longing.

Zeno: An ancient Greek philosopher, either Zeno of Elea (ca. 490–ca. 430 BCE) or Zeno of Citium (334–262 BCE), here quoted from Diogenes Laertius, a later Greco-Roman biographer of the third century CE.

lupines: Also "lupins," a flowering legume related to peas, eaten and used in medicine around the Mediterranean in antiquity and the Middle Ages, but now just considered a pretty wildflower.

Platearius on Leprosy in Theory and Practice[10]

Platearius was a famous Salernitan physician in the twelfth century. His *Practica* was widely read through the later Middle Ages and survives in over 100 manuscripts. The work is organized, like most practical medical treatises of the later Middle Ages, in a head-to-toe fashion. It begins with eight kinds of fever that affect the entire body, followed by conditions which were believed to originate in the head: frenzy, lethargy, apoplexy, mania, and, of course, the head cold (catarrh). Leprosy is treated toward the end of the *Practica* as a disease of the skin and extremities. In the passages below, Platearius explains why he wrote this book, and in a later section he outlines the variety of skin conditions that were considered "leprosy" (*lepra*) during the High Middle Ages. While we might now consider some of these conditions as actual examples of Hansen's Disease (the preferred modern name for leprosy), others could have been any number of other skin problems.

ℰ

[Prologue]

He plays the part of a friend who agrees to the just requests of his friends, therefore the just request of friends must be transferred quickly to the outcome, lest it seem that affection has grown cold through leisure. For this reason, I, Platearius, agreeing with your prayers, most dear friends, have proposed to quickly describe the causes, signs, and cures of diseases, so that the desired result follows on your labor and your discretion may bring forth glory and honor for me. Nor do I propose to pursue the causes, signs, and cures of diseases in every little detail, both because the wide variety of certain words would disturb the fruits [of this task], and because all of these things have been sufficiently demonstrated in different works by other people. Therefore I happily obey and will pursue the proposed work for you, my companions, nor will I say every single thing which I might manage to say about every disease, but rather only those things which I have learned better by experience, those which I have been accustomed to use more frequently, and those which God has granted the desired result through my hand. Therefore let us begin with the *febris ephemera*....

---

10   Victoria Recio Muñoz, *La Practica de Plateario: Edición crítica, traducción y estudio,* Edizione Nazionale "La Scuola Medica Salernitana" 7 (Florence, 2016), 126, 776–80. Original translation by the editor of this volume.

Chapter 64: Leprosy

Leprosy is a corruption which is produced by the production of corresponding humors. It appears from the ingestion of melancholic foods such as lentils, donkey meat, etc., from choleric foods such as eating foods every day with lots of garlic, pepper, etc., from corrupt foods and those in contact with corruption such as infected pork, impure wine, etc., from corrupt air and infected air, by coming into contact with a leper, from the first sexual intercourse with a woman who has been with a leper, sometimes from birth itself, as when a person is born of corrupt semen, is nourished with impure blood or also when conception takes place during menstruation.

When the spirit is infected by any of these causes or when the humors are corrupted, there appears an impurity of the limbs and a corruption of the body and, therefore, leprosy. There are four types of leprosy: *elephantia* from natural melancholy, *leonina* from bile, *allopicia* from blood, *tiria* from phlegm.

In *elephantia* the eyes grow round, the eyelids are deformed, the nostrils grow narrow, the voice become raspy, small and hard swellings develop on the body, of which the small surfaces have no feelings, the nails grow large and unequal.

In *leonina* the eyes also grow round, but they swell with an inflammation of the veins and are made yellowish-red and move violently. The nose also becomes sharper, they suffer from acute hoarseness, the gums corrode, sometimes blood is expelled with the urine, the skin becomes rough and cracks, eyebrows fall out, erysipelas and dermatosis arise and when either case becomes chronic, the extremities dissolve.

In *allopicia* the eyebrows fall out entirely and the eyelids swell, for which reason it is called *allopicia*, because the patients lose their hair like *allopes*, that is, foxes. The eyes grow inflamed and turn violently red, red pustules develop on the face and sometimes all over the body, from which blood and pus flow, the nose grows large, smelling becomes difficult, the breath reeks, the cheeks swell, blood flows from the gums and there is quite a lot of blood in the urine.

In *tiria* soft swellings develop, the skin grows soft and turns pale, and water sprinkled on it does not adhere. White blisters appear, the nose is blocked, and the voice becomes raspy.

I must admit that all types of leprosy are incurable and especially *leonina* and *allopicia*. However, when the patient's disposition to suffer leprosy appears, he can be saved from future danger. But when the disease is already confirmed, the patient can be made comfortable and preserved from greater suffering in the future.

DOCUMENT 68:

Guy de Chauliac's Personal Experience with the Black Death[11]

The French surgeon Guy de Chauliac (ca. 1300–68) is one of the few medieval
commentators on the Black Death of whom we can say with assurance that
he had personal experience with the disease as both physician and patient. In
this passage from his *Chirurgia Magna*, "Great Surgery," written during the
second wave of the pandemic in 1360–63, Guy describes the epidemiology
and potential causes of the first wave of plague that hit Italy in 1348, as well as
giving an account of his own sickness. See Documents 77 and 78, pp. 232–35,
for more passages from this work specifically on surgery.

ev

Arrival of the Great Mortality

Interior swellings, especially those occurring in the principal members, are
dangerous. We saw this clearly in that great and unheard of mortality which
appeared while we were in Avignon in the year of the Lord 1348, in the sixth
year of the pontificate of Lord Clement VI, in whose service I, although
unworthy, was then active, and by his grace. May it not be displeasing if I
describe it, for the sake of its marvelous nature and as foresight because it
might happen again.

The aforesaid mortality began for us in the month of January and lasted
seven months. It had two kinds: the first lasted for two months, with a
continuous fever and the spitting of blood, and the people died within
three days; the second lasted for the rest of the time, also with a continuous
fever and swellings and carbuncles in the external parts, particularly in the
armpits and groin, and they died within five days.

It was of such a contagious nature, especially the one accompanied by
the spitting of blood, that one person caught it from another not only by
standing close to another but even by looking at them. It was so great that
people died without servants and were buried without priests. Father did not
visit his son, nor the son his father. Charity was dead, all hope thrown down.

And I call it the "great mortality" because it seemingly took over the
entire world. But it had begun in the Orient and thus, taking aim at the
world, crossed over to us in the West. It was so great that scarcely a quarter
of all people remained. And it is unheard of, because we have read about
that [disease] from the city of Craton and in Palestine and others in the

---

11   Guy de Chauliac, *Inventarium sive Chirurgia Magna*, edited by Michael R. McVaugh, 2 vols. (E.J.
    Brill, 1997), Vol. 1, 117–19. Original translation by the editor of this volume.

Epidemics which occurred in the time of Hippocrates, and the one which happened according to a subject people of the Romans in the book *De euchima*, in the time of Galen, and one in the city of Rome in the time of Gregory. There was none so great, because those had not occupied more than a single region, this one the whole world. Those were in some way treatable, this not at all.

It was useless and shameful for doctors, because they did not dare to visit patients for fear of being infected, and when they did make a visit they accomplished little and earned nothing, for all who were sick died, excepting a few towards the end, who managed to escape after their buboes had burst.

Many were uncertain what caused this great mortality. In some parts, people believed that Jews had poisoned the world, and so they murdered them. In some places, [people believed that it was the] disabled poor and the people chased them off; in others, the nobles, and therefore they could not go about the world. At last it came to such a point that guards were established in cities and towns, and they allowed nobody to enter unless they were well known. If they found any powders or ointments, they forced the people to swallow them, fearing they were poisons. Yet whatever people were saying, the truth is that there was a twofold cause of this mortality, one a universal agent, the other a particular patient. The universal agent was the disposition of a certain greater conjunction of three higher bodies—Saturn, Jupiter, and Mars—which occurred in the year of the Lord 1345, on the 24th of March, in the 19th degree of Aquarius. Greater conjunctions, as I have said in the book I wrote on astrology, signify marvelous, powerful and terrible events, such as changes in kingship, the arrival of prophets, and great mortalities, and these events follow the disposition of the nature of the signs and their aspects under which they occur.

Therefore it was no marvel if that great conjunction signified a marvelous and terrible mortality, because it was not only a sign of greater events, but rather seemingly of the greatest. Because [the conjunction] was in a human sign, it indicated a loss beyond human nature; and because the sign was fixed, it signified a long duration. For it began in the Orient a little after the conjunction and last to this day in **fifteenth year in the West**. It impressed so great a shape on the air and in other elements that—just as a magnet moves iron—so that [conjunction] moved heavy, burnt, and poisonous humors, and gathered internally, causing abscesses. From these there followed continuous fevers and bloody spit at the start, while the shape [of this disease] was powerful and confounded nature. Afterwards, when the disease had subsided, nature was not so confounded, and [the body] expelled [the humors] as far as it was able to the exterior parts, especially to the armpits and groin, and caused buboes and other swellings, in such a way that the external swellings were the effects of internal abscesses.

fifteenth year in the West: Guy is writing in 1360, 15 years after the conjunction.

The particular and "patient" cause was the disposition of bodies, such as **cacochimia**, weakening, and obstruction. Because of this laborers and those living badly died. As a cure, people labored for prevention before the attack, and in care during the event. As prevention there was nothing better than to flee the region before the infection and to purge oneself with aloe pills, to let blood with **phlebotomy**, to improve the air with fire, to comfort the heart with **theriac** and fruit and perfumes, to animate the humors with Armenian bole, and to resist putrefaction with acidic things. As a cure, people used, evacuations, electuaries, and cordial syrups. External abscesses were ripened with figs and cooked onions, crushed and mixed with yeast and butter, after which they opened and could be cured by the treatment for ulcers. The carbuncles were treated by cupping, scarification, and **cautery**. And I, for the sake of avoiding infamy, did not dare to flee; but, always fearful, I strengthened myself as well as I could with the aforesaid remedies. Nevertheless, toward the end of the mortality I incurred a continuous fever with swellings in the groin. I lay sick, apparently, for six weeks, and I was in such great danger that all my friends believed that I would die. Yet my swelling ripened and was cured, as I have said, and I escaped, with God's permission.

cacochimia: Cacochymy in English, the term for a body overcome with bad or excess humors, and thus diseased in multiple ways.

phlebotomy: Cutting into a vein for the purpose of medical bloodletting, usually to balance the humors. Also called venesection.

theriac: One of the most famous compound medicines of Antiquity and the Middle Ages, supposedly made of viper's flesh and numerous other exotic and expensive ingredients. It was believed to be a cure-all and every good apothecary, even up to the nineteenth century, carried a stock of theriac.

cautery: The application of burning hot irons to specific points on the body in order to modify the internal humors, such as through the removal or destruction of bad humors, or the creation of pus in the burn, which medieval physicians frequently saw as a beneficial sign.

The writings of al-Rāzī, Usamah ibn Munqidh (Documents 56–58, pp. 168–76), and other medical authors provide us models of physicians acting with authority. Those physicians were almost always male in the Mediterranean cultures. A rare exception of a medieval woman acting publicly as a physician was one Trota, or Trocta, of Salerno in the early twelfth century. She was apparently one of numerous Salernitan women (*mulieres Salernitanae*) known for their medical skill. The physician and anatomist Copho of Salerno (Document 79, pp. 238–39) mentions these women with respect. Trota wrote her own medical works, including a *Practica* very like the work of the same title by Platearius (Document 67, pp. 201–02). She is also credited with an ensemble called the *Trotula* ("little Trota"), a compilation of three short works on women's health. Trota did not write the *Trotula*, but it was probably compiled by other (mostly male) physicians from her ideas and teaching. Until the recent and transformative scholarship of Monica Green, historians believed that "Trotula" was the name of a person, not a book composed in her honor. In another passage from the *Trotula* (Document 83, pp. 245–46), the author(s) provide a detailed description of treatments for retained period (amenorrhea). These include the full range of treatments available in the twelfth century: bloodletting, pills, medicated baths, fumigations, and applications. The learned authority of this work is demonstrated by the citations of Galen and the prescription of complex antidotes with Greek names.

Europe during the High Middle Ages went through startling transformations in every area of study, not just in medicine. Formal education grew dramatically as schools in cathedrals and large churches were revived or established, replacing the older monastic schools, and teachers established their own private schools in large cities. By the end of the twelfth century, groups of schools and masters in Bologna, Paris, and Oxford were coalescing into the first universities. A university education in the arts and philosophy included basic medical theory, which was considered part of a well-rounded education. In the later Middle Ages several universities established formal, graduate faculties of medicine. The three short sources in Document 70 display the formalization of a standard medical curriculum in Western Europe. Each source outlines the most important medical books at that time and together they show the movement of formal medical education from monasteries to established universities. They include a list of recommended medical books written ca. 1100 (70a), most of which were recent products of Salerno and Montecassino; a ca. 1200 description of the favorite books on medicine taught in the schools of Paris at that time (70b); and a required reading list from the 1270s for students pursuing a degree in medicine at the University of Paris (70c).

In later medieval Europe, medical authority could be gained from a university education or by popular support, but it could also be granted by a political authority. Some European states and larger cities sought to control and license medical practitioners, as part of a broader move on the part of political leaders in the later Middle Ages to control and protect their entire populations. This process began in southern Italy, near the medical center of Salerno, and especially in the Kingdom of Naples. Document 71 reproduces two licenses to practice surgery (rather than internal medicine) within the lands of Naples. The first was granted by Robert I the Wise, King of Naples, to Bernard of Casale Santa Maria in 1330, and then by Queen Joanna I (Giovanna) to Maria Incarnata of Naples in 1343.

Some medieval women, such as Trota of Salerno (see Document 69 and Document 83, pp. 208–09 and 245–46) and Maria Incarnata, were allowed to practice medicine or surgery, but by the later Middle Ages women were being driven out of the profession by university-educated male physicians, many of whom were also ordained clerics. One such woman physician was Jacoba Felicie. She was the defendant in a trial in 1322, in which the dean and masters of the Faculty of Medicine in the University of Paris charged that she was illegally practicing medicine. This came at the time when university faculties, including that of medicine, were attempting to control more strictly the practice of their respective arts, be it teaching, law, medicine, or theology. Document 72 is a record of that trial and includes the arguments of the dean and masters of the Faculty of Medicine, and of Jacoba herself.

Trota of Salerno as a Medical Master[12]

Trota was a physician and author in Salerno during the early twelfth century, one of numerous Salernitan women (*mulieres Salernitanae*) known for their healing skills. She wrote her own medical works, including a *Practica* like that by Platearius (Document 67, pp. 201–02), in which she provides learned treatments for every kind of ailment. She is known best, albeit indirectly, through a medical work written (probably by men) in her honor called the *Trotula* ("little Trota"), containing three works on women's health: *Book on the Conditions of Women*, *On Treatments for Women*, *On Women's Cosmetics*. In the passage below from *On Treatments for Women* Trota herself appears as a female master (*magistra*) of medicine. It records an episode when she was called on to treat a young woman with painful "wind" in her womb. The description of Trota is important for understanding how women healers could be viewed in the twelfth century: she was summoned "as if she were a master of this craft" (*uocata fuit quasi magistra operis*), the implication being that women normally were not masters of medicine at this time. *Magistra* is the feminine form of *magister*, and the latter was a title usually reserved only for scholars who had attended cathedral schools or universities, where women were not allowed.

ev

On Wind Entering into the Womb

There are some women who take wind up through the vagina, which is received in the right or left part of the womb and generates such a great windiness that the women appear as if they are suffering from a rupture or intestinal pain. In just such a case, it happened that Trota was summoned—as if she were a master of this craft—when a certain young woman was going to be operated on because she seemed to be suffering from a rupture on account of this sort of windiness. Trota was very much amazed at this, and she made the woman come into her house so that she could understand the cause of her illness in private. She then understood that the pain was not from a rupture or swelling of the womb, but that it was borne from windiness. She thus ordered a bath to be made for her in which mallow and pellitory were heated, and she placed her in it, where she rubbed her limbs often and thoroughly to soften them. She ordered the young woman

---

12 *The Trotula: A Medieval Compendium of Women's Medicine*, edited by Monica H. Green (U of Pennsylvania P, 2001), 126–28. Original translation by the editor of this volume.

to remain in the bath for a long time, and after she got out, Trota made a plaster for her from radish juice and barley flour. She applied all of this, warmed, for a little bit, to consume the windiness, and again caused her to sit in the aforesaid bath. She thus remained cured.

Medical Education in High Medieval Europe (Three Accounts)

The three short documents below demonstrate the formalization of medical education in the High Middle Ages. Document 70a comes from a medical manuscript made in Italy around 1100. The main text in this manuscript is a copy of the herbal of Macer Floridus (Document 73, pp. 221–23), followed by several short texts useful to a practitioner of a Hippocratic medicine: a poem on weights and measures, a note on the division of hours, a catalogue of medical books, followed by several dozen brief medical recipes. The book catalogue reflects the latest medical texts coming out of Salerno and Montecassino; about half of these are translations by Constantine the African (see Documents 62 and 66, pp. 188–90 and pp. 199–200). The list in Document 70b was written about a century later (ca. 1200) by the English monk Alexander Nequam. He described the works read in Paris in theology, medicine, and other fields, while he was a student there in the 1170s. The list is almost identical to Document 70a, but the works are now being taught in lectures beginning with the foundational *Isagoge* of Johannitius (Document 52, pp. 153–57). Document 70c provides more detailed instructions for candidates pursuing a license in medicine from the new Faculty of Medicine in the University of Paris in the 1270s. In that list, the work called *Art of Medicine* is not a single book, but a set curriculum of medical texts which was used by European medical students for over half a millennium (ca. 1150–1700). This curriculum, later known as the *Articella*, first included the *Isagoge* of Johannitius, Hippocratic *Aphorisms*, Hippocratic *Prognostics*, *Urines* of Theophilus, and *Pulses* of Philaretus. By the later twelfth century the *Articella* usually included the *Tegni* of Galen as well, in the translation of Constantine the African. The surgeon Guy de Chauliac invokes the authority of the *Tegni* several times in Documents 77–78, pp. 232–35.

(a) "These Are the Books of Medicine," Italy, ca. 1100[13]

These are the books of medicine: *Pantegni, Megategni, Book of Fevers, Liber aureus, Passionarius, Antidotarium, Book of Eyes, Book of Coitus, Book of Urines of Isaac, Book of Melancholy, Dioscorides, Book on Interior Parts, Tereoperica, Gynaecia of Cleopatra, Universal and Particular Diets.*

---

13 Vatican City, Biblioteca Apostolica Vaticana, ms Vat. Lat. 2825, fol. 31r. Original translation by the editor of this volume.

(b) Alexander Nequam, Medical Reading List from Paris in the Twelfth Century[14]

Anyone who desires to study medicine, which is very useful for the sons of Adam, should attend lectures on Johannitius, both the *Aphorisms* and the *Prognostics* of Hippocrates, the *Tegni* of Galen, and the *Pantegni*. Galen is the author of this book but Constantine is the translator. He should also read the *Universal and Particular Diets* of Isaac, his *Book of Urines*, the *Viaticum* of Constantine, with the *Book of Urines*, Dioscorides and Macer in which the nature of herbs is treated, and the books of Alexander.

(c) University of Paris Medical License Reading List, 1270s[15]

This is the format for **bachelors** seeking to be licensed in medicine. In the first place the master under whom the bachelor is [studying] ought to make an oath to the chancellor, in the presence of the masters summoned for this, concerning the suitability of the bachelor seeking the license. He ought to prove the time he spent hearing [lectures] through at least two witnesses: he ought to have attended lectures for five and a half years if he held a chair or was licensed in the Arts, or for six years if he was not chaired or licensed. The format for hearing [lectures] on the books is such: he ought to have heard the *Art of Medicine* twice in ordinary lectures and once in cursory lectures, except for the *Urines* of Theophilus, which it is sufficient to have heard once in ordinary or cursory lecture; the *Viaticum* twice in ordinary lecture; the other books of Isaac once in ordinary and twice in cursory, except the *Particular Diets*, which it is sufficient to have heard in cursory or ordinary lecture; the *Antidotarium of Nicholas* once. The *Verses of Gilles* are not part of this format. Likewise he ought to have read one book of the *Theorica* and another of the *Practica*. He must swear by this, but if anyone should be convicted of perjury or lying, he can be driven out of the licentiate.

bachelors: Students in medieval universities who have achieved the first, preliminary degree in the liberal arts and are seeking further education as masters in the fields of philosophy, theology, law, or medicine. We still use the same terminology in our Bachelor's and Master's degrees.

---

14 Alexander Nequam, *Sacerdos ad Altare*, in *Studies in the History of Mediaeval Science*, edited by Charles Homer Haskins (Harvard UP, 1927), 374–75. Original translation by the editor of this volume.

15 *Chartularium Universitatis Parisiensis*, edited by H. Denifle and E. Chatelain (Paris, 1889–97), Vol. 1, no. 543, p. 517. Original translation by the editor of this volume.

DOCUMENT 71:

Licenses for Male and Female Surgeons in Medieval Naples[16]

The two documents translated below are licenses for a man and a woman to practice surgery in the Kingdom of Naples. Robert I the Wise, King of Naples, granted the first to Bernard of Casale Santa Maria in 1330, and Queen Joanna I (Giovanna) granted the second to Maria Incarnata of Naples in 1343. Both licenses are for the practice of surgery, rather than internal medicine (see Documents 76–78, pp. 229–35 for more on surgery); the latter required literacy and a university education, which neither of these recipients had.

e

For Bernard of Casale Santa Maria (1330)

Robert, etc. To all those throughout the provinces of Terra di Lavoro and the county of Molise and Capitanata who will be reading these letters, his faithful servants, greetings, etc. Physicians were established by divine ordinance for curing sick bodies; so that they might be proficient in the office of practical procedures, they are selected by the provident science of medicine by approved physicians who assist Us. Clearly, master Bernard of Casale Santa Maria Gilberto, an unlettered surgeon, our faithful and lawful servant, born from a faithful family [as acknowledged] by public written testimony of the municipality of Bagnoli (whose praiseworthy testimony Our Court receives), and whom we had diligently examined by our surgeons, is found to be experienced in [treating] bones. Hence, having first received from him the customary oath of fidelity sworn on the holy Gospels of God, that according to the traditions of this same art he will practice faithfully. We are led to concede to him by the tenor of the present letters a license to treat and to practice on bones broken in the arms and legs, throughout the whole of the above-said provinces. We order, by Our faith, that this same Bernard shall be free to treat and to practice on the aforementioned broken bones of the arms and legs throughout each of the lands and places of these provinces to the honor and fidelity of Us and Our heirs and to the utility of Our faithful servants of these same parts, no impediment or obstacle withstanding. Given at Naples by John Grillo of Salerno, etc., the year of Our Lord 1330, the ninth day of May, of the thirteenth indiction, the twenty-first year of our reign.

---

16 *Medieval Italy: Texts in Translation*, edited by Katherine L. Jansen, Joanna Drell, and Frances Andrews (U of Pennsylvania P, 2009), Part 75, translated by Monica H. Green from Raffaele Calvanico, *Fonti per la storia della medicina e della chirurgia per il regno di Napoli nel periodo angioino (a. 1273–1410)* (Naples: L'Arte Tipografica, 1962), 323–25.

On Surgery. For Maria Incarnata (1343)

Giovanna, etc. To all those throughout the province of Terra di Lavoro and the County of Molise who will be reading these letters both now and in the future, her faithful servants, greetings, etc. With respect to the public weal as it relates to the upstanding women of Our [kingdom], we have been attentive and we are mindful in how much modesty recommends honesty of morals. Clearly, Maria Incarnata of Naples, our faithful servant, present in our Court has proved that [she] is competent in the principal exercise of surgery, in the treatment of wounds and **apostemes**. She conducts herself with circumspect judgement in such cases, because of which she has supplicated Our Highness most attentively that we might deign to concede to her a license to practice on diseases or conditions of this kind. Because, therefore, by trustworthy testimony presented to Our Court, it is clearly found that the above-said Maria is faithful and comes from a worthy family and, having been examined by our surgeons, she is found to be competent in treating the above-said illnesses. Although it should be alien to female propriety to be interested in the affairs of men lest they rush into things abusive of matronly shame and for this reason they risk the sin of forbidden transgression, [nevertheless] because the office of medicine is expediently conceded to women by an unspoken rule of law, it being noted that females, by their honesty of character, are more suited than men to treat sick women, especially in their own diseases, We, having first received from this same Maria the customary oath of fidelity sworn on the Gospels and [the promise] that she will faithfully treat [patients] according to the traditions of this art, impart to her a license to treat and to practice on the mentioned afflictions throughout the whole of the above-said Principality, by the counsel and consent of the glorious lady, **Lady Sancia**, by the grace of God Queen of Jerusalem and Sicily, reverend lady mother, administrator and our principal governor, and by the public authority of our other administrators. Therefore by our faith from the counsel and assent of the above-mentioned, we command that it be ordered that in so far as this same Maria treats and practices on the above-said diseases through the whole of the above-said Principality, to the honor and our faith and of our heirs and the utility of the faithful of these same provinces, you should permit her freely [to do so], posing no impediment or obstruction to her. Given at Naples by Adenulf Cumano of Naples, professor of civil law, Vice Protonotarius of the Kingdom of Sicily, in the year of Our Lord 1343, the seventh day of May of the eleventh indiction, the first year of our reign.

apostemes: A swelling or abscess filled with pus.

Lady Sancia: Queen of Naples (r. 1309–43) as wife of Robert the Wise. Her family claimed the throne of Jerusalem even though Christians had lost the city over a century earlier.

A Woman Physician on Trial in Medieval Paris, 1322[17]

> Jacoba Felicie was a practicing physician in fourteenth-century Paris, but her
> right to diagnose patients and prescribe internal medicines was challenged on
> the basis of her gender by the dean and masters of the Faculty of Medicine in
> the University of Paris. The following document is the transcript of her trial
> in 1322 for practicing medicine illegally. The dean and masters of medicine
> argued that only male, university-trained scholars of medicine should be
> allowed to practice the full range of scholarly medicine. The passage below
> contains Jacoba's defense, but her arguments were rejected.

⁓

October 6–23, 1322. Paris
The Questioning of Witnesses against Jacoba Felicie

... The Dean and masters of the Faculty of Medicine, teaching in Paris,
intend to prove against Lady Jacoba Felicie, the accused: 1) That the said
Jacoba visited in Paris and in the suburbs many sick people suffering from
grave sicknesses, very often observing their urines both jointly and separately,
taking their pulse, and palpating and holding their bodies and limbs. 2) That
after this observation of urine and touching she said and is accustomed to
say to those patients: "I will heal you, God willing, if you have faith in me,"
making an agreement with them for their cure and receiving money from
them. 3) That after the agreement was made between the accused and the
patients or their friends for the purpose of curing them of their internal
sickness and wound or abscess appearing on the outside of the bodies of
the aforesaid patients, the accused very often visited and still visits the
aforesaid patients constantly and continuously, observing their urines in
the manner of physicians and doctors, taking their pulse, and touching
and holding their bodies and limbs. 4) Also that after these touches and
activities she gave and gives to the aforesaid patients syrups for drinking;
comforting, laxative, and digestive medicines, both liquid and not liquid;
aromatic herbs, and other drinks, which they take and drink and have drunk
very often by the mouth in the presence of the accused, while she prescribes
and gives these medicines. 5) That she very often exercised and exercises the
practical duties of medicine, in relation to the aforesaid activities, continually in Paris and in its suburbs, she practiced and practices this from day

---

17 *Chartularium Universitatis Parisiensis*, edited by H. Denifle and E. Chatelain, 4 vols. (Delalain,
1889–97), Vol. II, 255–67. Original translation by the editor of this volume.

to day, even though she was not approved in any solemn study at Paris or elsewhere, and she has no license from the **Chancellor** of the Church of Paris and from the aforesaid Dean and masters. 6) That she does this against the laws, by which she was not and is not approved, and because she had been warned by the mandate of the venerable Official of Paris under pain of excommunication and sixty Parisian pounds, that she no longer should practice, as described above, in Paris and in the suburbs, and she should act under the aforesaid penalties, since she was neither licensed nor approved by the aforesaid Chancellor, Dean or masters.... 7) That the accused, having spurned this warning and prohibition made to her, she was neither approved nor licensed by the said persons in Paris, as stated above, and she practiced and practices in Paris and its suburbs, incessantly visiting the sick, giving them the aforesaid potions, observing their urine, and diagnosing (as she believes) their infirmity, as was said.

The Interrogation Follows

The witnesses were led forth and interrogated by the Dean, etc., against the said Jacoba Felicie, in what neighborhood of Paris she visited the sick, or in what part of the suburbs. Likewise whether they had been present during the aforesaid visit. Likewise, concerning Article 1, if they had seen the said Jacoba take the pulse of the patients for the purpose of diagnosing their sicknesses and not otherwise. Likewise, concerning Article 2, if they had seen the said Jacoba inspect urines, and if she was doing this for the purpose that she recognize their infirmities. Likewise if they had been present when she said the words contained in the said article, namely: "I will heal you," etc. Likewise if they had seen her haggle over taking a payment for her to cure the said infirmities. Likewise, concerning Article 3, whether they were standing with her during the visit to the aforesaid patients and during the inspection of urines and taking of their pulses. Likewise, concerning Article 4, if they had been present for the giving of syrups, and of what sort of quality were the said syrups, and whether digestives or laxatives, etc., whether she had done the aforesaid things like a practitioner of surgery or of medicine. Likewise, concerning Article 5, if they were with her on any day when she practices in the city of Paris and suburbs, and whether they knew that she was not approved in any general area of study in Paris or elsewhere, and if they had seen her at Montpellier. Likewise, concerning Article 6, whether they had seen her warned, and if [they knew that] the Official of Paris was able to warn these sort of practitioners and to fine them in this case with a pecuniary punishment. Likewise, concerning the last Article, whether they had seen her after this warning was made to continue the practice of medicine, and in what neighborhood of Paris and the suburbs, and who had

Chancellor: The Chancellor was a senior clerical officer in the cathedral of Notre Dame (here called "the Church of Paris"), who held the authority to grant degrees ("licenses") to approved students in the University of Paris.

been visited by her for the diagnosis of infirmities, and if she had done this for the sake of money, for the sake of friendship or for free, and if she had done these things, whether she called herself a surgeon or doctor [*medicam*].

Thereafter follows the interrogations of seven Parisians, all of whom paid Jacoba Felicie for medical care. They include men and women, craftsmen, merchants, and nobles.

[Jacoba's Defense]

... These are the reasons which the aforesaid Jacoba states and proposes in judgment before you, Master Johannes de Villa Parisiaca, clerk, in the case prepared on the part of the venerable men the Dean and masters in the art of Medicine against the noblewoman Lady Jacoba Felicie, that is, against the aforesaid Dean and masters, and their procuration, petition, warning, and prohibition, which they have prepared against her or are endeavoring to use for the purpose of a defense of this sort.

... The aforesaid Jacoba states that if a statute, decree, warning, prohibition, and excommunication had ever been made, which the said Dean and masters endeavored to use against her, this was done at one time merely because of and against idiots and foolish ignoramuses, those unlearned in the medical art and totally ignorant of its precepts who usurp the practical office of medicine. The said Jacoba is exempt from their number, as she is expert in the art of medicine and instructed in the precepts of the said art. On account of this, the aforesaid statute, decree, warning, prohibition, and excommunication do not bind her, nor are they able to find her, because with the cause ceasing, the effect ceases, and the aforesaid vices cease in her.

Likewise, the aforesaid statute and decree, etc., had been issued on account of and against the aforesaid idiots and usurping fools, and those who were at that time exercising the practical office of medicine in Paris, who were now dead or so decrepit and ancient that they are not able to exercise the said office, as appears from the tenor of the aforesaid statute and decree, etc., which had been made one hundred and two years in the past [i.e., 1220], at which time Jacoba was not alive nor did she exist in nature afterwards for another sixty years. Rather, she is young, that is to say thirty years old or nearly, as can be seen from her appearance.

Likewise, in the aforesaid statute and decree, etc. are contained these words: "we have established and decreed," and these indicate a time which is greater and longer and more ancient than the said one hundred and two years, of which quite ancient time there is no confidence, for the said words presuppose that the statute and decree had been issued at another time than the writing of those letters....

Likewise, it is better and more honorable and equitable that a woman who is wise and expert in the art visit another sick woman, and observe and inquire into the secrets of her nature and her hidden parts, than for a woman, to whom it is not permitted to see such things, to inquire after them, nor to touch the hands, breasts, stomach and feet, etc., of women. Rather, a man ought to shun and flee from the secrets of women and the hidden matters associated with them as much as possible. In previous times, a woman would rather die, than to reveal the secrets of her infirmity to a man, on account of the honor of the female sex and on account of the shame she would suffer by revealing them. And for these reasons many women and even men died from their sicknesses, not wishing to have doctors lest they should see their secrets.

Likewise, let it be supposed, without prejudice, that it were a bad thing for a women to visit, cure, and investigate [a patient], as had been said, etc., yet it is less bad that a woman who is wise, discerning, and expert in the aforesaid matters should have practiced and still practices the aforesaid, because patients of either sex, who have not dared to reveal the said private parts to a man, did not wish that they should die. Now it is the case that the laws say that lesser evils should be permitted that greater ones can be avoided. Therefore since the said Jacoba is an expert in the art of medicine, it is better and ought to be permitted to her that she visit [patients] to exercise the practical office [of medicine], than for the patients to die, especially because she cures and heals everyone in her care....

PART 9

Medical Practice in the High Middle Ages (ca. 1000–1400 CE)

The medical theories of humoralism and complexion, described in Part 8, were used to explain and reinvent medical practice during the High Middle Ages. Two of the most common medical practices in this period were, just as today, the prescription of drugs and the practice of surgery. Examples of how these medical traditions were transformed by humoralism are reproduced in the first two sections of this chapter. These medical practices could be applied more or less equally to men and women, but obstetrics and gynecology were of course intended primarily for women. Sources in the final section of the chapter show how these medical fields also were transformed by the revival of learned medicine in high medieval Europe.

HERBALISM AND PHARMACOLOGY (DOCUMENTS 73–75)

In the eleventh century somebody (most likely a French cleric named Odo of Meung) composed a new herbal in Latin verse under the pseudonym "Macer Floridus" ("Flowery Macer"), after the first century CE Roman poet Aemilius Macer. This herbal, *De viribus herbarum* (Document 73, "On the powers of herbs"), was clear, short, and memorable—the perfect vehicle for learning the basics of medical herbalism—and it thus became one of the most popular herbals for nearly half a millennium, ca. 1100–1600. Macer's *De viribus herbarum* was hugely popular, being copied hundreds of times in manuscript and adapted into Latin and vernacular prose, incorporated into encyclopedias, or rewritten by other poets. Such is the case with Henry, Archdeacon of Huntingdon (ca. 1088–1157), who wrote his own lengthy herbal in verse, the *Anglicanus ortus* ("The English Garden") around the year 1140. Henry, however, was a far better poet than Macer, and he demonstrates how herbal knowledge could be made even more entertaining and memorable, as seen in his account of the herb mandrake in Document 74.

Whereas the herbals of Macer Floridus and Henry of Huntingdon drew primarily on medical knowledge that had been circulating since the later Roman Empire, new pharmacological works appeared in the twelfth century which rebuilt the science of pharmacology in imitation of the newly rationalized medicine of Salerno and Montecassino. One such work was the *Circa instans* of Matthaeus Platearius (Document 75), who was probably related to the Platearius who wrote the *Practica* in Document 67 (pp. 201–02). *Circa instans* is a catalogue of the medicinal attributes of single herbs, spices, and minerals. Its usual name comes from its incipit, i.e., the two opening words in Latin, but it was also often called "The Book of Simple Medicines," because a "simple" was a medicine made from just one ingredient, as opposed to an "antidote" compounded of multiple substances. *Circa instans* would become, along with the *Antidotarium Nicolai* ("Antidotary of Nicholas [of Salerno]"), one of the most popular pharmacological manuals of the later Middle Ages. He draws on the full Arabic-Galenic system of medical theory, based on humors and complexion as described in Parts 7 and 8.

DOCUMENT 73:

Macer Floridus, *On the Virtues of Herbs*[1]

During the eleventh and twelfth centuries many technical subjects, such as law, theology, and medicine, were presented in Latin verse to help students and practitioners learn and remember them better. One of the most popular medical works of the High Middle Ages was the verse herbal *De viribus herbarum* ("On the powers of herbs") by "Macer Floridus," a pseudonym, probably for a French cleric named Odo of Meung. At least two hundred manuscripts survive of the Latin original, and it was translated into every European vernacular as well as Hebrew before 1500, while also being the first herbal in print (1471). Macer wrote poems on the medicinal virtues of 65 plants native to Europe and the Mediterranean and of 12 exotic spices from Asia and the Indian Ocean basin. Below are examples from each of those sections: the common Eurasian herb artemisia (mugwort) and black pepper, the most popular Asian spice in medieval cuisine. Spices like pepper were used in both cooking and medicine.

℮

Artemisia

Since I will be singing the powers of herbs,
I think it fitting to place first the mother of herbs,
To which the Greeks gave the name *Artemisia*.
Diana is said to have discovered its virtue first,
She who is called Artemis in Greek, and from her
The herb takes its name, because she is called its finder.
It especially cures women's diseases:
Taking a decoction of it provokes menstruation,
And it does this if the vulva is often washed with it,
Or if, raw, it is mixed and ground with wine, and drunk,
Or if the powdered green herb is bound to the belly at night.
It forces out a fetus by merely a drink or as a suppository,
And it dissolved uterine lumps and banishes tumors.
In a drink, it stimulates urine and forces out stones,
And when drunk often with wine helps the jaundiced.
Pliny praises the application of this, mixed with lard,
For scrofula and orders that one take it, ground, with wine.

---

1 *Macer Floridus de Viribus Herbarum...*, edited by L. Choulant (Leipzig, 1832). Original translation by the editor of this volume.

If an overdose of opium harms someone, this herb
Helps greatly if it is mixed with wine and drunk.
Some affirm that whoever should taste it
Cannot be sickened by any harmful medicine,
And that no wild animal is able to bite him.
Its root, when hung from the neck with brambles,
Is said to ward off all harmful frogs,
And a drink of its juice with wine also is beneficial.
If the fresh herb is ground and preserved in wine must,
It renders the mind medicinal for the aforesaid diseases.
The flavor and odor of that wine are very pleasing;
When drunk, it strengthens the stomach, cleans the vitals,
And they affirm that it is useful for many other conditions.

Pepper

To the several common herbs already mentioned in my song,
I now will try to add those spices which the custom of selling
Has made known to almost everyone,
And, first, I think I need to plead the powers of Pepper,
Which Cooking makes more famous than Medicine.
Pepper is claimed to be of virtue dry and hot,
And the third degree is granted it in both of these.
It has three varieties: white and long and black,
But because only two are known to physicians,
I will say certain things known to me about the black variety.
When taken raw or cooked, or mixed with honey,
It will help the stomach or liver's digestive power.
It cures poisonous bites, takes away distaste,
Often hinders various problems of the torso,
And the regular fever which is apt to cause a chill
Is checked, if Pepper is taken before the fever's tremor.
It settles gripes when drunk with laurel berries
Or well-ground laurel leaves, and with tepid wine.
When mixed with hardened pitch and applied,
It removes scrofulous sores; it is fittingly mixed with [medicines]
Which are accustomed to purge the eyes of a fearful mist.
When mixed with **soda** in a plaster, it removes blotches.
Mix and grind an equal weight of pepper with the powder
Of burnt human excrement and apply it thus to cankers:
The experts say nothing is more useful than this powder.
No one is able to enumerate all the powers of Pepper,

soda: Native soda, *nitrum* in Latin, a natural form of sodium salts or alum.

For almost every medicine requires Pepper,
And it is apt to be added to many precious antidotes.
Hence I think it is that so few praises are said about Pepper alone,
Because it is worthy of praise as part of countless medicines.

DOCUMENT 74:

Henry of Huntingdon, Herbalism in *The English Garden*[2]

Like Macer Floridus, Henry, Archdeacon of Huntingdon (ca. 1088–1157), wrote his own herbal in Latin verse, the *Anglicanus ortus* ("The English Garden") around the year 1140. He rewrote Macer's herbal but added nearly 100 other herbs and spices in his own creative style. The *Anglicanus ortus* was not as popular as Macer's herbal, probably because it was too long, and not as immediately useful for a practicing herbalist because he added little medical information that could not be found from Macer or the works of Constantine the African (Documents 62, pp. 188–90 and 66, pp. 199–200). The example below, mandrake, is now well known from the Harry Potter books and movies: the plant was believed to be shaped like a person, to come in male and female varieties, and to kill people who heard its scream when unearthed.

૮ઃ

Mandrake, *Mandragora officinarum* L.

Illustrious Mandrake stands high in an elevated bed,
rightly found in the foremost place. If our garden did not
have these, perhaps England would lack these riches:
Since it is the prince of herbs, as man is over animals,
this prince in body imitates the body of the other prince,
to wit, the feet with feet, leg with leg, genitals with genitals,
hips with hips, chest with chest, throat with throat,
and head and hands by the shape of head and hands.
In place of digits the feet and hands are made of roots,
but observe that the hairs found on the head grow out as leaves:
they grow anew each spring and fade away at summer's end.
And as many relate (though I don't assert this firmly),
if someone digs it up and should hear it being torn
from its mother's womb, that man may die just like the herb.
They dig around it and, running away, bind a dog
to the mandrake's body; the hungry dog goes for some food
placed far away; the herb is plucked and the dog is slain.

You know what this is and of what kind. Learn what it can do:
Mandrake juice is said and known to calm

---

2   Henry of Huntingdon, *Anglicanus Ortus: A Verse Herbal of the Twelfth Century*, edited and translated by Winston Black (Pontifical Institute of Mediaeval Studies Press, 2012), 2.1, 130–33.

a headache, if the forehead is rubbed with it.
Add the aforesaid juice to oil of **nard**;
by pouring it in you can cure an earache.
Beyond that, take a pinch from the right foot
and a pinch from the right hand; make a powder
from them and then grind the powder into wine;
when drunk for seven days it can, with quick result,
cure gout; to be sure, it will alleviate the swelling.
This likewise will recall pulled tendons to each other,
if an ounce of the splendid body is obtained, if you pound
it with oil once obtained, if you rub it on once pounded;
this ointment is able to help strained limbs.
Also, take a pinch from the mandrake's body;
it is good to give this in warm water to an epileptic,
and thus you can remove the suffering of rabies.
A little patch of it is hung from a sick man's neck,
and some claim that like this it is better than an amulet.

nard: Spikenard or muskroot, the aromatic essential oil of *Nardostachys jatamansi*, an Asian member of the valerian family.

DOCUMENT 75:

Matthaeus Platearius: Rationalizing Simple and Compound Medicines[3]

The *Circa instans* of Matthaeus Platearius (fl.1150) is a catalogue of the medicinal attributes of single herbs, spices, and minerals, so named from the first two words of the Latin prologue, *Circa instans* (roughly "Getting down to business"). It represents a new type of pharmacological work appearing in the twelfth century that applied Arabic-Galenic medical concepts of humoralism, complexion, elemental qualities, and treatment by contraries to traditional herbalism. In his prologue Matthaeus Platearius discusses the nature of both "simple" medicines, based on just one herb or spice, and "compound" medicines composed of multiple ingredients. Like the herbals of Macer Floridus and Henry of Huntingdon (see Documents 73–74), his book describes just "simple" medicines, but he does so in a manner that would help a physician or apothecary better prepare effective compound medicines.

ev

Prologue

Here begins the book on medicinal simples according the Platearius, called *Circa instans*. Getting down to business, our plan concerns simple medicines. A simple medicine is the sort which is produced by nature, such as cloves, nutmeg, and the like, or that which, although it is modified by some artifice, is not mixed with another medicine, such as tamarinds, which are broken up by artifice after their skins are removed, or aloes, which is made from the juice of an herb, cooked down in an artificial manner.

But here's a question, and not an idle one: Why were compound medicines invented, when every virtue which is in compound medicines can be found in simple medicines? Medicine, they say, was invented because of disease. But the cause of every disease happens either from the abundance of humors, or from their emptiness, either from the flux or debility of virtues, either from the **change of qualities** or from the **dissolution of continuity**. A simple medicine can be found which can dissolve abundance and restore emptiness, restrain a flux, comfort a weakness, halt a change, or consolidate a loosening.

change of qualities: When a body goes from cold to hot, or vice versa, and moist to dry, or vice versa.

dissolution of continuity: A technical term for any significant, usually negative, change or break in the composition of a part of the body. It usually means a wound or an ulcer. The term usually appears as "solution of continuity" in English translation. See Document 77, p. 000.

---

3   *Das Arzneidrogenbuch "Circa instans" in einer Fassung des XIII. Jahrhunderts aus der Universitätsbibliothek Erlangen*, edited by Hans Wölfel (A. Preilipper, 1939), 1. Original translation by the editor of this volume.

Solution

There exist multiple reasons for compound medicines, namely, 1) the violence of the disease, 2) the opposition of diseases, 3) the contrary disposition of members, 4) the nobility of a member, or 5) the violence of diseases:

1. The violence of a disease, such as leprosy, apoplexy, and epilepsy, which is either scarcely or in no way cured by simple medicines. And so it was fitting that compound medicines appear, so that after their virtue is increased from the simples, the curing of a violent illness may be made easier.

2. When opposing diseases occur in the same body, such as the fever *leucoflegmantia*, it is necessary to have a medicine composed of hot and cold, so that it is able to block contrary diseases with contrary properties, for one and the same simple medicine cannot be found which is endowed with contrary qualities.

3. When members, however, are affected by contrary qualities, such as the stomach by cold and the liver by hot, a compound medicine was necessary, so that it can also alternate the contrary qualities with the contrary qualities of the members.

4. And also the nobility of a member, such as, perhaps, when the liver is suffering *sclerosis* a compound medicine was necessary, since the dissolution of the superfluous humor occurs with a hot medicine, and the comforting of the noble member with an astringent medicine. For a hot medicine, only dissolving, weakens the noble member, unless it is comforted with astringency.

5. And a violent medicine, such as scammony or hellebore and the like simply ought not to be given, unless other medicines are mixed with them to alter their violence.

In my treatment of every simple medicine, the complexion of the subject must be offered first; consequently whether it is a tree or fruit, herb, root, or flower, seed, leaf, or stone, juice or some other thing; and after that how many forms of it there are, and how they are made, and in what place they are found; also, what form is better, how they are adulterated and known to be adulterated, and how the subject is able to be preserved, and what virtues they have, and how they ought to be shown. This treatment of spices will be fulfilled according to the order of the alphabet.

leucoflegmantia: A condition in medieval medicine characterized by excess phlegm, producing subcutaneous water retention (dropsy) and white, bloated skin. In the case of a "leucophlegmatic" fever, the physician must use cold substances to counter the fever, but hot substances to counter the cold phlegm.

Many of the Arabic and Latin works reproduced in Parts 7 and 8 reflect the revived Galenic medical theory of the Middle Ages and its applications in medicines and dietary regimen. But another significant aspect of medieval Islamicate medicine was surgery, as seen in the work of Albucasis, the Latin rendering of Abu al-Qasim Khalaf ibn al-'Abbas al-Zahrawi al-Ansari. He was an Arabic physician and author who died around 1013 CE. His most famous work, *On Surgery and Surgical Instruments* (Document 76), treats subjects such as cautery, treating incision and perforation, and setting bones and dislocations. Note that these are mostly superficial surgical procedures, for almost no surgeon in Europe or Islamicate lands practiced internal surgery.

Albucasis's *On Surgery* was translated into Latin by Gerard of Cremona (ca. 1114–87) and became one of the primary textbooks on learned surgery in later medieval Europe. An original European work on surgery that was influenced by Albucasis and other translations from the Arabic was *Chirurgia Magna*, "Great Surgery," of Guy de Chauliac, whom we met above discussing plague (Document 68). In the passage from this same work in Document 77 Guy applies contemporary medical theory and technology to the treatment of wounds. Guy belonged to a growing number of literate surgeons in the later Middle Ages who wanted to elevate their craft to a learned science on par with the Hippocratic-Galenic medicine taught in the universities. Guy describes the nature of wounds in highly technical and learned language inspired by the theories of classical and Arabic medicine. In another passage from his "Great Surgery" (Document 78) he presents his opinion on how a surgeon should train and present himself professionally. Guy quotes often from Greek and Arabic medical authorities to prove his standing alongside "Hippocratic" physicians.

DOCUMENT 76:

Learned Surgery: Albucasis on the Treatment of Cataracts[4]

Albucasis (Abu al-Qasim Khalaf ibn al-'Abbas al-Zahrawi al-Ansari) was an Arabic physician and author who died around 1013 CE. His most famous work, *On Surgery and Surgical Instruments*, is divided into three books: on cautery; on incision and perforation; on setting bones and dislocations. Albucasis and other Arabic physicians are famous for their surgical treatment for eye cataracts, a process called "couching," described in the passages below. But credit for couching is also due to the ancient Romans, who had mastered this process. The main source for Albucasis's chapter on cataract surgery (II.23) is Celsus's *De medicina* (see Documents 15, p. 55, and 22, pp. 76–77), although many of the details seem to come from his own experience or observation.

ع

I.12. On Cautery in Cataract of the Eye

When by those signs I have mentioned in the relevant section there is brought to your notice the beginning of a cataract of the eye, start with draughts for the patient such as shall cleanse his head; and guard him from all humidities. Make him also sweat for some days, fasting, in the bath. Then tell him to have his head shaved; and burn him with one cauterization in the middle of the head; then cauterize him with two burns on the temples if the cataract is beginning in both eyes; or on the one side only if it is in one eye. And with the cautery cut all the subcutaneous veins and arteries; and let the cauterizations be long, across the breadth of the temples. Beware of hemorrhage; if you see any, stanch it straight away with any means you can. We shall deal later with the method of extraction and cutting out of arteries, and provision against hemorrhage.[5] Two strong cauterizations are sometimes made on the back of the neck below the two bones.

II.23. On the Couching of Cataract

We have already mentioned in the appropriate section the varieties of cataract and those in which depression is useful, in full detail; so you may take it accurately from there. You should cause the patient to sit down cross-legged

---

4   *Albucasis on Surgery and Instruments: A Definitive Edition of the Arabic Text with English Translation and Commentary*, edited and translated by M.S. Spink and G.L. Lewis (The Wellcome Institute, 1973), 42, 252–56.

5   He does this later in Book I, ch. 56, "On cauterization in hemorrhage arising from a cut artery."

before you, facing the light in full sun, and firmly bind up his sound eye. Then lift up his eyelid with your left hand, if it be the left eye in which the humor is; or with the right hand if it be the right eye. Then take the couching needle in your right hand if it be the left eye; or in your left hand if it be the right eye. Then put the tip of the needle near the corona, about the thickness of a probe away, onto the white of the eye itself, on the side of the lesser canthus. Then thrust the needle firmly in, at the same time rotating it with your hand, until it penetrates the white of the eye, and you feel that the needle has reached something empty. The depth the needle goes in should measure as the distance from the pupil to the edge of the iris, which is the corona of the eye; you will see the metal in the pupil itself because of the transparency of the corneal tunic. Then put the needle up to the place containing the humor; then press the point downwards time after time. If the humor comes down at once, the patient will at once see whatever his vision is opened upon while the needle is still in his eye. Then let him rest a little while; and if the humor goes back up again depress it a second time without taking the needle out. When it stays down firmly and does not come back again, gently draw the needle out, twisting it ever so slowly with your hand. Then dissolve a little pure rock-salt in water and wash the eyeball with the solution; then apply all over the outer aspect of the eye carded linen or wool moistened with oil of roses and egg-white, and bandage it up together with the sound eye. Now we and our contemporaries apply pounded cumin with the egg-white.

But if the couching needle does not serve, failing to enter the eye on account of the hardness (for there are some whose eyes are hard indeed), you should take the scalpel called *al-barid* figured thus.[6] With this make a perforation in the conjunctiva only, not piercing any further; for that is only to make a little entrance for the needle. And then thrust in the needle as we said before.

At the end of your operation, prepare a solidly-built bed on which the patient may lie on his back, in a dark room; and keep him from all movement or coughing. And prescribe such a diet for him as will relax his system; neither let him move his head to right or to left. Let the bandage remain in the same position till the third day. Then loosen it in the same dark room and make trial of his sight, putting before him objects to be seen; then replace the bandage till the seventh day. You should not do this at the time of treatment nor immediately after the perforation by the needle; but on the contrary you should avoid it, for intensive use of the eye causes a rapid

---

6   Albucasis provided diagrams of many of the specialized surgical implements he describes. In most manuscripts of his works, especially in the Latin European versions, these diagrams have become mere decorations and look nothing like the intended instruments.

ascent of the humor. But if an abscess occur you should unbandage the eye before the seventh day and restore it to health by those methods that allay swelling. When it has subsided, allow him free sight, putting over his face a dark veil beneath which his vision may be exercised for a few days while he is still in the dark room. Then let him come out of the room gradually and take up the exercise of his business. But you should know that in the case of a depression of a cataract the student cannot manage without having seen that operation performed several times; then he may perform it himself. I have heard that a certain Iraqi has said that in Iraq he makes a hollow needle by which the humor is sucked out. In our land I have never seen anyone do it in this fashion, nor have I read of it described in any books of the **Ancients**; perhaps it is newly invented.

Ancients: Albucasis likely means the writings of ancient Greek and Roman physicians, especially Hippocrates and Galen, but he could also refer to more recent Arabic authors of the ninth century CE, like Hunayn ibn Ishāq (see Document 52, p. 153).

Applying Medical Theory to Wound Treatment: Guy de Chauliac[7]

> Guy de Chauliac was one of the leading surgeons in Europe, famed for elevating the craft of surgery to a learned science on par with Hippocratic medicine. In the passage below from his *Chirurgia Magna* ("Great Surgery"), Guy describes the nature of wounds in technical and learned language, and supports his arguments with citations from the best of classical and Arabic medicine as taught in the universities.

ev

Book III, Chapter 1: Introduction on Wounds and the Solution of Continuity

solution of continuity: A technical term for any significant, usually negative, change or break in the composition of a part of the body. It usually means a wound or an ulcer.

Averroes: The Latin name for the Muslim Andalusian philosopher Ibn Rushd (1126–98 CE). He wrote commentaries on nearly every work by Aristotle, and most of these were translated into Latin during the thirteenth century, so that he became better known to Christian Europeans than to Muslims. He also wrote several medical treatises, including the *al-Kulliyat fi al-Tibb* ("General Principles of Medicine"), which was known in Europe by its Latin title *Colliget*.

Tegni: The Latin title of Galen's most important medical work, the *Art of Medicine* (*Techne iatrike*), translated by Constantine the African from an Arabic version. This work is not to be confused with Constantine's *Pantegni* (Document 62, pp. 188–90) or the collection of medical works known as the *Articella* or *Art of Medicine*.

A wound is a "**solution of continuity**," recent, bloody, without putrefaction, made in the soft parts. "Solution of continuity" is given there as that kind of disease, in the first book on sickness and symptoms, which is common to the simple and composite parts of the body. Nevertheless it is more properly present in the simple parts than the composite, according to **Averroes** in the second and third parts of the *Colliget*, since in those parts an account of continuity is more truly discerned. The remaining parts [of the definition] are provided for the sake of differentiation (namely "recent, bloody, without putrefaction") to differentiate it from an ulcer, which does occur with putrefaction. "In the soft parts" is provided to differentiate from fractures, which pertain to the solid limbs. It was according to this general division of body parts that Johannitius said that surgery was twofold, either in the flesh or in the bone, for he understood flesh to be the muscles, nerves, and veins, which the new commentator on the third part of the *Tegni* included under the soft and middle parts of the body....

Treatment. The common goal for every "solution of continuity" is unity, as in the third part of the *Tegni*. This is the first indication known to all from the essence of a disease, which orders remedies to reject the contrary with its own contrary. To be sure, this first and general goal is accomplished by two things: by Nature, as the principal agent, operating under its own powers and with suitable nourishment; and by the doctor, as a servant, operating with five goals, subalternate to each other: The first requires the removal of foreign objects if there are any among the divided parts; the second is to join together the divided parts to each other; the third is to preserve the parts

---

7 Guy de Chauliac, *Inventarium sive Chirurgia Magna*, edited by Michael R. McVaugh, 2 vols. (E.J. Brill, 1997), Vol. I, 134, 141. Original translation by the editor of this volume.

once they are set back in place and brought together as one; the fourth to conserve and preserve the substance of the body part; the fifth teaches how to correct complications.

The First Goal, which is to remove foreign objects. The first thing to be completed is that the wound be opened, if it is not open and something foreign is found between the parts, such as a fragment of bone puncturing the separated parts or something lodged in, like an arrow or another foreign object like a thorn. And if it is sufficiently opened, the object should be removed and extracted gently and without pain using the fingers or forceps or *tenaculae* or with some other instrument which you yourself devise.

[Guy proceeds to describe a selection of tools for extracting arrows and other foreign bodies lodged in wounds. This passage is frequently accompanied by images of the tools in the manuscripts and early printed editions of the text.]

tenaculae: Among the most important surgical tools, both in the past and today. They are used for delicate grasping of objects and small body parts.

DOCUMENT 78:

Training and Decorum for the Learned Surgeon[8]

We met Guy de Chauliac above writing about the Black Death (Document 68, pp. 203–05) and wound treatment (Document 77), but here he presents his opinion on how a surgeon should train and present himself professionally. This was a major concern for some surgeons, who generally were not granted the academic or social standing held by Hippocratic physicians. Guy establishes his authority as a learned medical practitioner by quoting often from ancient Greek and medieval Arabic medical authorities.

℮

Life is brief ... difficult: This aphorism and others are found above in the Hippocratic *Aphorisms*, Document 10, pp. 39–41.

Arnald: Arnaldus (Arnau) de Vilanova (ca. 1240–1311) was a Spanish physician, medical author, and religious reformer. He was the master of the Paris faculty of medicine 1291–99, but he was later condemned for heretical beliefs and his religious works burnt. Later in the Middle Ages he gained a reputation as an alchemist, astrologer, and magician.

medicine: Guy uses the word *physica* here for medicine, which usually implied the learned and theoretical medicine of Hippocrates and Galen, as opposed to *medicina*, which applied more broadly to any form of healing.

naturals and non-naturals and those against nature: On these terms, see the *Isagoge* of Johannitius in Document 52, pp. 153–57.

Introduction: This work could be Galen's *Tegni* ("Art") or more likely the *Isagoge* of Johannitius (Document 52, pp. 153–57), which was not by Galen but served as an introduction to Galenic medical theory.

Let us return to our purpose, and establish the conditions required of any surgeon who wishes to skillfully exercise this manner and form of operating on the human body. It is fitting not only that a surgeon himself exhibits those conditions which Hippocrates, our leader in all good things, summed up with a certain subtle reasoning in the first part of his *Aphorisms*—"**Life is brief, and art is long, experience is deceiving, and the judgment difficult**"—but also what things the patient and the assistants ought to exhibit and how he ought to display himself externally. These are the fourfold conditions which are accepted here, according to **Arnald**, that most eloquent Latin translator: there are some things which are required in the surgeon, some in the patient, some in the assistants, but others in external events.

There are four conditions required of a surgeon: first, that he be literate; second, that he be trained; third, that he be clever; fourth, that he be pleasant. Therefore, in the first place, it is required that the surgeon be literate, not only in the principle of surgery but also of **medicine**, both in theory and in practice. As to theory, it is fitting that he understands the **naturals and non-naturals and those against nature**. First, it is fitting that he understands the naturals, especially anatomy, for without that nothing can be accomplished in surgery, as will be made clear below. He should also understand complexion, for it is right to vary medicines according to the diversity in the nature of bodies....

As to practice, it is fitting that he knows how to devise a diet and prescribe drugs, for without these skills surgery, which is the third instrument of medicine, is not complete. Concerning this, Galen said in his ***Introduction***: Just as pharmacy needs diet and surgery, so also surgery needs diet and pharmacy....

---

8   *Inventarium sive Chirurgia Magna*, Vol. 1, 8–9. Original translation by the editor of this volume.

Second, I said that he ought to be trained and he should observe others operating. So, according to the wise **Avenzoar**: It is fitting for every doctor first to understand, and then to have skill and experience...

Third, that he be clever and possess good judgment and memory, and **Haly Rodoan** says this about the Third book of the *Tegni*: It is fitting that a doctor have a good memory, good judgment, good dexterity, good eyesight and a balanced intellect, with a fitting shape, as (for example) graceful fingers, strong hands which do not shake, bright eyes, and so on.

Fourth, I said he should be agreeable; bold in times of safety, cautious in times of danger; that he avoids bad practices. Let him be dear to his patients, benevolent to his friends, careful in his prognostications. He should be chaste, sober, dutiful, and merciful; neither greedy nor extortionate, he should accept moderate payments according to his labor and the patient's means, the quality of the outcome and his own social standing.

Avenzoar: The Latin name for the Spanish Muslim physician and surgeon Ibn Zuhr (1094–1162 CE), whose "Book on Simplification concerning Therapeutics and Diet" was translated into Latin and Hebrew.

Haly Rodoan: The Latin European corruption of the name of Ali ibn Ridwan (988–1061 CE), an Egyptian physician and astrologer. He wrote a commentary on Galen's *Tegni* (also known as the *Ars Parva*), which Guy de Chauliac knew in the Latin translation of Gerard of Cremona.

Some of the earliest medical documents focus on the treatment of women, especially when it concerns conception and childbirth (see Document 1, p. 14, and Documents 29 and 30, pp. 93–95). During the High Middle Ages, gynecology again became an independent area of medicine and women's anatomy was also recognized as distinct from men's. Anatomy, more than almost any field related to medicine, disappeared in the Early Middle Ages in Europe and would not revive until the later eleventh or early twelfth century (an important exception is the gynecological manual *Gynaecia* written by Muscio in the sixth century CE based on the writings of Soranus of Ephesus; see Document 30, pp. 94–95). Like so many other facets of medical revival in the High Middle Ages, the revival of gynecology texts also occurred in southern Italy, perhaps in or near Salerno, influenced by a vigorous anatomical tradition in the Islamicate world. Dissection of human bodies, however, was frowned upon (if not forbidden explicitly) by all three monotheistic religions. Anatomy, therefore, had to be learned entirely from books or from human analogues, such as pigs or apes, which were believed to be composed much like humans internally. European physicians would not regularly dissect humans and make new advances in human anatomy until the fourteenth century.

The text, *Anatomia Porci* ("Anatomy of a Pig"), is credited to Copho, a physician apparently working and teaching in Salerno in the early twelfth century. He may have known the real Trota (see Documents 69, pp. 208–09, and 83, pp. 245–46), as she used some of his writings, and he used some of hers. Copho walks the reader through the dissection of a pig and its major organs, with the understanding that this knowledge could be transferred to human patients. Document 79 includes the introduction to this work, which defines anatomy, and a later section on the anatomy of the uterus. Copho objectifies the woman and her uterus, describing it both as a bilge pump for removing women's "superfluities" and as a "field ... cultivated that it may bear fruit." He refers to midwives, from whom he apparently obtained some of his knowledge of birth and the fetus.

In the decades around 1100 the learned medicine of the Arabic world and Salerno moved into Western and Northern Europe, most likely through the literary and religious networks connecting monastic houses. Several English medieval manuscripts from this time include a short text called *De urinis mulierum*, "On Women's Urines" (Document 80). It provides a brief guide for interpreting the urine of women and its diagnostic significance according to its appearance and placement in a urine glass. Women's bodies and their urine are defined according to marriage and childbearing: urine appears different depending on whether a woman is married, menstruating, or pregnant. This fixation on pregnancy is also clearly relevant in writings on contraception. Birth control was (and often still is) considered sinful in the monotheistic religions, but there are nonetheless many recipes for contraception and abortion surviving in medieval texts, written by both women and men. The Muslim physician Avicenna (see Documents 53 and 54, pp. 158–64) briefly outlined in his *Canon* fourteen methods for preventing conception (Document 81), but prefaces them with a statement meant to appease religious authorities that this should be done only in case of medical necessity.

Basic medical knowledge, founded on the ideas of Hippocrates and Galen, became part of a well-rounded education in the twelfth and thirteenth centuries (see the medical curricula in Document 70, pp. 210–11). This form of education was available primarily to men but some women (especially those dedicated to religion as nuns) did also gain significant medical learning. One of the greatest intellects of the twelfth century was St. Hildegard, Abbess of Bingen (1098–1179), who is known equally as a religious prophet, poet, composer, and natural philosopher. She is credited with two medical works, the *Physica* and *Causae et Curae* (*Causes and Cures*). In both of them she incorporates her medicine with a deep knowledge of nature and Christian theology, as seen in her description of menstruation in *Causes and Cures* (Document 82).

Much of the medical literature by medieval Jews was written in classical Arabic or Judaeo-Arabic, like the treatises of Maimonides (Document 55, pp. 165–67), rather than in Hebrew, which language was reserved for religious topics. But in the twelfth century, many Jews left the Islamicate culture of Spain (Al-Andalus) because the Almohad rulers began to persecute non-Muslims. A growing number of non-religious works were translated into or written in Hebrew by European Jews. One of the most important translators worked in southern France and took the biblical pseudonym Doeg ha-Edomi (Doeg the Edomite), but his real identity is unknown. He translated at least 24 medical works, including those by Constantine the African and from the *Trotula*, into Hebrew. Doeg helped start a later medieval tradition of Hebrew-language medical works in Europe, like the treatise on childbirth in Document 84 from the fourteenth or fifteenth century. It is based on the *Gynaecia* of Muscio, itself based on the *Gynaecology* of Soranus (Document 30, pp. 94–95), or perhaps the Hebrew rendition of Muscio, *Sefer ha-Toledet*, made by Doeg.

DOCUMENT 79:

Anatomy of the Uterus, Learned from a Pig[9]

Anatomia Porci ("Anatomy of a Pig"), is credited to Copho, a physician in Salerno in the early twelfth century. Copho walks the reader through the anatomical dissection of a pig and its major organs, with the understanding that this knowledge could be transferred to human patients. Below are reproduced the introduction to this work, which defines anatomy, and a later section on the anatomy of the uterus, which gives Copho the opportunity to explain his understanding of conception. The ovaries are imagined as "testicles" producing "the female seed," which joins with the male seed to form the fetus. The identification of separate egg and sperm in human reproduction were theorized in the 1670s but only observed in humans in 1827.

Because the structure of the internal parts of the human body was almost wholly unknown, the ancient physicians, and especially Galen, undertook to display the positions of the internal organs by the dissection of brutes. Although some animals, such as monkeys, are found to resemble ourselves in external form, there are none so like us internally as the pig, and for this reason we are about to conduct an anatomy upon this animal.

The term *anatomy* signifies "correct division," which is performed as follows: place the pig on its back and incise its throat in the middle. The first thing which presents itself is the vocal organ, which is bound on the right and the left by certain nerves, called *motivi*. Also there come to the vocal organ, from below, certain nerves which are called *reversivi*, because after proceeding from the brain to the lung they return to the vocal organ, by which means it is moved in producing the voice. Nearby these are fleshy masses called *pharynges*, and the same term is applied to swelling of these structures. There are also in this region large glands in which humors collect and cause tumor of the throat. At the base of the tongue arise two passages, namely, the *trachea arteria*, through which air passes to the lung, and the esophagus, through which food is transported to the stomach. The *trachea arteria* lies in front of the esophagus, and upon it there is a certain cartilage known as epiglottis, which at times closes to prevent the entrance of food and drink, opening at other times to allow entrance and exit of air....

---

9   *Anatomia Porci*, in George Washington Corner, *Anatomical Texts of the Early Middle Ages* (Washington, DC, 1927), 51–53.

It is next necessary to discuss the anatomy of the uterus. It must be recognized that nature has contrived this organ in women in order that whatever superfluities are generated during the course of the month may be sent to this organ as if to form the bilge-water of the whole body; this is the nature of the menses which women have. This organ is also nature's field, which is cultivated that it may bear fruit; in which, when seed is sown, it remains as on good ground and through the cooperative action of natural warmth, and the mediation of vital spirits, it becomes implanted like a germinating seed, and sends out twigs through certain roots or mouths by which it is attached to the uterus, and through which nutriment is delivered to it and to the future foetus. Thus, later on, by the action of the bodily forces (as I have often told you, you may recall) the foetus-to-be is generated and augmented. The uterus is located above the intestine; above its neck is the bladder, and under it the **longaon**. Below is the vulva. Next cut the uterus through the middle of its *os*; you will find two testicles attached above it, by which the female seed is transmitted to the uterus and joins the male seed to form the foetus. The uterus has seven cells, and if the animal is pregnant, you will find the foetuses in these chambers. Over them you will find a kind of tunic, like a chemise, which is called **secundine**. This is broken when the foetus strives for exit. It is attached to the uterus and to the foetus by veins which run in it, and it carries nutriment to the uterus and to the foetus. These openings by which the foetus is attached are called *cotyledons*. There is also a large channel, called umbilicus, which is broken (near the uterus when the foetus is delivered; midwives tie it) at a distance of four fingers from the foetus. When it is ligatured this causes *phlegmons* of the umbilicus.

longaon: The sixth and final segment of the intestines, according to medieval anatomists, which terminates with the anus.

secundine: Literally, the "followings," or the placenta, which becomes the afterbirth.

DOCUMENT 80:
A Brief Medieval Guide to Uroscopy of Women[10]

Sources 61–65 above show the central role of uroscopy, or the diagnostic analysis of urine, in medieval medicine, and it also played a key role in high medieval obstetrics. The short text *De urinis mulierum*, "On Women's Urines," found in several twelfth-century manuscripts, provides a brief but systematic guide for interpreting the urine of women and its significance according to its appearance and placement in a urine glass (see Documents 64 and 65, pp. 195–96).

e

Here begins the *Urines of Women*. Virgin girls make a bright urine, as well as a clear urine. The urine of a married woman is cloudy and the man's semen appears in the bottom of the glass. The urine of a menstruating woman seems to be bloody. The urine of a pregnant woman, if she is in the first month or second or third, is cloudy at the top, and white in the ***hypostasis*** (sediment), and the **urine** is very clear. The urine of a pregnant woman who has already had four months is clear and has the color of wine and a white *hypostasis*. The lower part is fatty and shining.

hypostasis: Sediment at the bottom of a jar of urine. The Latin author retained the Greek term *hypostasis*, meaning the sediment at the bottom of the urine flask, indicating that the language of Hippocrates and Galen still possessed terminology that was untranslatable in Latin.

urine: This is the urine in the middle of the glass, as opposed to the *hypostasis* sediment at the bottom.

---

10 Monica H. Green, "Making Motherhood in Medieval England: The Evidence from Medicine," in *Motherhood, Religion, and Society in Medieval Europe, 400–1400,* edited by Lesley Smith and Conrad Leyser (Routledge, 2016), 179. Original translation by the editor of this volume.

DOCUMENT 81:

Contraceptives in the *Canon* of Avicenna[11]

In this excerpt from his *Canon of Medicine*, the Muslim physician Avicenna (ca. 980–1037 CE, see Documents 53 and 54, pp. 158–64) outlines 14 methods for preventing conception, but prefaces them with a statement that this should be done only in medical necessity. Some of the methods involve the cooperation of both the man and woman before or during sexual intercourse, but other methods rely on the woman inserting or ingesting an herbal remedy without necessarily informing her sexual partner.

e

Prohibiting Conception

The physician finds it necessary to prevent conception in small women, in whom it would be dangerous to have a childbirth on account of a diseased womb or from a weakness in the insides. A heavy fetus causes clefts in the internal area to such a degree that urine passes involuntarily and she is unable to retain it full term. Among the measures for this situation are: [1] One should anticipate those times for coitus which are favorable for conception to occur as we have said [elsewhere]; [2] One should separate before mixing the two seeds; [3] The woman should raise immediately after coitus, jump backwards from seven to nine times forcefully so that the sperm may come out; [4] Another way is for the woman to sneeze; [5] And also one can add slippery things to the sperm so that it is dissipated. Along these lines one could put **pitch** and white lead on the penis before coitus and afterwards put [in the vagina] pulp of pomegranate and alum; [6] Or one could put cabbage flowers or seed as a suppository near the time of the cleaning period and before coitus; [7] Using the same procedure before and after coitus one can use the same dipped in pitch or submerged in a decoction of pennyroyal; [8] Or, as a suppository willow leaves after the menstruation period and by its property [as a contraceptive] it is especially good if [the pad] is submerged with water in which willow leaves have soaked. And the same [purpose] is obtained by [9] equal parts of colocynth pulp, mandrake, iron dross, sulfur, scammony, and cabbage seeds, collected, mixed with pitch and inserted. [10] And inserting pepper after coitus prohibits conception, and [11] so does a suppository of elephant's dung by itself or in **fumigations** at the times mentioned previously; [12] and it is also useful to drink three *okas*

pitch: Natural bitumen or asphalt, or possibly a resin derived from plants.

fumigations: The burning of a substance for medical purposes, to be inhaled or brought up into the uterus.

okas: A liquid measurement roughly equivalent to the imperial pint.

---

11 John M. Riddle, *Contraception and Abortion from the Ancient World to the Renaissance* (Harvard UP, 1992), 128–29.

of an infusion of sweet basil, for it prevents conception. [13] If the penis, particularly the glans, is anointed with sweet oil before coitus, conception is prevented; [14] likewise, the leaves of bindweed prevent conception if a woman inserts them after the menstruation begins.

DOCUMENT 82:

St. Hildegard of Bingen: A Moralized Explanation of Menstruation[12]

St. Hildegard, Abbess of Bingen (1098–1179) is credited with two medical
works, the *Physica* and *Causae et Curae* (*Causes and Cures*), in which she
blends medicine with a deep knowledge of nature and Christian theology.
In this excerpt from *Causes and Cures* Hildegard explains why women
menstruate partly in religious terms, as a punishment for Original Sin, but
also in humoral terms. Compare her descriptions of menstrual blood with the
analysis of women's urine above in Document 80 and note how both texts
define women primarily in terms of virginity and motherhood.

~

Why Is There Menstruation?

When an influx of desire entered Eve, all of her veins were opened with a
flow of blood. For this reason every woman has in her body storms of blood,
so that she retains or pours forth drops of her own blood, in the likeness of
the shrinking and overflowing of the moon, and all her body parts, which
are united by the veins, open up. For just as the moon waxes and wanes, so
the blood and humors are purged at the time of menstruation in women,
otherwise she could not survive, because she is moister than a man, and
would fall victim to a serious disease.

Modesty, however, is the enclosure of integrity in a virgin, because she
has evaded the activity of a man, ignorant of that same activity, and therefore
menstrual blood in a virgin is bloodier than in a woman, since the virgin is
still closed. For after a virgin is corrupted, then she has more **darkness** in
her menstrual blood, because it is corrupted, than she had before, when she
was a virgin. And when a girl is still in her virginal integrity, her periods
are then in her like drops from her veins. But after she is corrupted, then
the drops flow out like a stream, because they are released through a man's
activity, and therefore they are like a stream, since the veins have been loos-
ened in that activity. When the enclosure of integrity in a virgin is broken,
that breaking sends forth blood. For a woman is created in such a way, that
she ought to seize and retain a man's semen with her blood, and therefore
she is also weak and cold and the humors in her are sickly. For this reason
she would always be sick, if it were not that her blood is purged through
menstruation, just as food in a pot is purged when it throws up froth.

darkness: Hildegard's
word is *livor*, which means
a bluish-black color, like a
bruise, but also can mean
"envy." For Hildegard,
medical *livor* is much more
than just a color. It also has
a spiritual or moral sense of
decay, shame, and sin.

---

12 *Hildegardis Causae et Curae*, edited by Paulus Kaiser (Leipzig, 1903), 102–03. Original translation by
the editor of this volume.

On the Corruption of Eve

All of the veins in a woman would have remained whole and healthy, if Eve had remained forever in Paradise. For when she, after agreeing with the serpent, looked upon it, her sight, which saw heavenly things, was snuffed out. And when she heard the serpent in their agreement, her hearing, which heard heavenly things, was blocked up. And with the taste of that apple, the splendor which gleamed all about her was shadowed. But just as sap begins in the root of a tree and reaches upward to all the branches of the tree, so also it is with a woman in her time of menstruation. For in that time of streaming blood, her veins, which contain the brain which hold the sight and hearing, are beaten about with the effusion of blood. And the veins, which support the neck and back and kidneys draw toward themselves the veins of the liver, intestines, and navel, and every single vein pours itself into another, just like the greenness of a tree causes the branches to turn green. And the veins, which support the kidneys, dissolve **that wheel** on which the kidneys are joined together, and they contract and retract it, just as the talons of some small bird, to be cut off, are contracted or released by their veins.

that wheel: This refers, it seems, to the network of veins, muscles, and ureters that attach the kidneys to the surrounding organs.

Trotula: Treating Retention of the Period in Medieval Italy[13]

> We first met Trota of Salerno and the work known as the *Trotula* above
> in Document 69, pp. 208–09. Here the author(s) of the *Trotula* provide
> a detailed description of treatments for retained period (amenorrhea).
> These include the full range of treatments available in the twelfth century:
> bloodletting, pills, medicated baths, fumigations, and the prescription of
> complex antidotes with Greek names.

℘

Retention of the Period

If the menses are deficient and women's body is overly thin, then bleed her
from the vein which is under the ankle of the foot, on the first day from
one foot, and on the following day from the other. The blood should be
extracted according to what her strength can handle, because in every illness we generally ought to be careful and respectful so that the patient is
not overly weakened. Galen told about a woman whose period had failed
for nine months, and she was constricted and overly thin throughout her
whole body, and her appetite had wholly failed. He drew her blood from
the aforesaid vein for three days, one pound from one foot on the first day,
one pound from the other foot on the second day, eight ounces from the
first foot on the third day, and so in a short time her color, warmth, and
usual bearing came back to her.

Very often women are constipated in the belly. In that case, prescribe five
pills of any suitable medicine. Then properly strengthen [the medicine] as
far as she is able to tolerate its strength, and give it to her. Bleed her then
from the *sophena*. Let her bathe, and after the bath she should have a drink
of calamint or catnip of mint, cooked in honey, but in such a way that it
contains eight parts water and a ninth of honey. The bath must be repeated
often, and after the bath she should drink one denarius of *diathesseron* or
two denarii with honey and water. *Diathesseron* is made from four spices,
namely mint or myrtle, gentian, birthwort, and laurel berries. Mix these
together at an equal weight, with cooked honey, and have her take this like
hierapigra or *hieralogodion*.

All diuretic remedies are beneficial for her, like fennel, spikenard, celery,
cumin, cowbane, caraway, parsley, and the like. All of the herbs together, or

sophena: The major vein
in each leg, extending from
the femur to below the
ankle. It is most likely the
same vein that is ordered
bled in the first paragraph
above.

diathesseron: A form of
the famous compound
medicine called theriac,
made of four main
ingredients (which is
the meaning of *dia-
thesseron*). It appears in the
popular twelfth-century
pharmaceutical manual
Antidotarium Nicolai.

**hierapigra or
hieralogodion:** Two
famous compound
medicines popularized by
the *Antidotarium Nicolai.*
Hierapigra (or *hiera picra*) in
particular was employed in
Western medicine until the
modern era. The preface
hiera- is Greek for "sacred"
and was applied to many
important remedies.

---

13 Monica H. Green, editor, *The Trotula: A Medieval Compendium of Women's Medicine* (U of
Pennsylvania P, 2001), 74–76. Original translation by the editor of this volume.

taken individually, are beneficial when cooked in wine or drunk with honey. Galen teaches that mugwort ground in wine and drunk is very good, or it helps when cooked and drunk in wine. Catnip, if drunk while in the bath, also helps, or when it is cooked in that bath. Or you can bind it on the belly, ground up when green, either below or above the navel, or cook it down in a pot, have the woman place a perforated chair over it, and have her sit on it, covered all around, letting the smoke ascend through a reed, so that the smoke can penetrate to her womb once it is taken up inside through the reed.

DOCUMENT 84:

A Medieval Hebrew Treatise on Difficult Births[14]

> The following treatise on childbirth was written in Hebrew during the fourteenth or fifteenth century. It is based on the *Gynaecia* of Muscio, itself an adaptation of the *Gynaecology* of Soranus (Document 30, pp. 94–95). It demonstrates all the hallmarks of learned medicine in the High Middle Ages: a medical condition is defined, the causes are explored, instructions are provided to the physician in recognizing symptoms and making a diagnosis, and only then are cures outlined (compare the *Practica* of Platearius, Document 67, pp. 201–02).

ᴄᴇ

On Difficulties of Birth. The birth can be natural, unnatural, or difficult— and for that reason it is especially worthwhile to examine the natural. The natural birth occurs most at the end of the seventh month or the ninth or the tenth. And the head should emerge first with the face downwards, and afterwards the neck, and after that the shoulder, and it should be that his hands will be alongside the body. The unnatural birth occurs when the legs emerge first, or the hands, or the sides. The difficult birth [is] when the foetus cannot emerge and tortures the mother and oppresses her—she will stand that anguish and that anxiety for a long time.

    The reason for anguished birth may be external or internal. The external reason may be extreme heat or extreme cold, or when the midwife is not wise, or when the uterus has been severely injured in its opening and was stitched up so that when the birth time arrived it could not widen. Or when the birth occurs at an unnatural time or when the mother suffers certain diseases in the abdomen. Or when she is very restrained.

    And if it is from internal reasons it may be because the girl became pregnant before she had her signs of maturity and her ways are narrow. Or when she is fat and the opening of the uterus is closed, or when the woman is spoiled and damaged, or when the foetus is very big and gross, or when he is thin and feeble and he cannot help himself. Or when the foetus is dead, or when his head is very big, or when he has two heads, or when there are twins, or when the birth is unnatural, or when it occurs before time, or when the woman is very old, or as a result of the uterus' diseases, or when

---

14 Ron Barkai, "A Medieval Hebrew Treatise on Obstetrics," *Medical History* 33 (1988), 96–119: 115–17. The bracketed words and phrases are original to Barkai's translation. I have removed his other editorial marks for ease of reading.

the uterus is little by nature and shrivelled, or the uterus is dry and empty of beneficent moisture.

The Signs. If his mother is strong, and the external reasons and the other well-known [reasons] will be shown [as not being the cause of a difficult labour], then it is a sign that the birth difficulty is caused by the placenta. And if it is due to the dying foetus, then the signs are severe pains around the navel, and slight fever, and a horrible expression, and a stinking smell, and stinking vapours rising, and the abdomen does not move, and the insomnia, and the other signs; all of them can be recognized from the patient's words.

Anticipation of diagnosis. When the pains are going downward and the breathing is regular, the birth will be easy. The male emerges with less anguish than the female; fat women suffer more during the birth than thin ones.

The cure or correction. When the birth time is approaching, the woman will have a bath in water with Indian aloe-tree, bish, aloe, sweet-violet, camomile, melilot, and after that will be anointed with sesame oil and sweet almond oil and hen's suet, and after that she will descend to a bath place, and when the birth time will be closer, she will eat little food but of good quality, such as fat hen soup, and will drink the fragrant wine. And after that, when the birth will be closer, and the thin membrane will be broken and some water emerges, she has to breathe forcefully and to massage forcefully downwards, because this kind of pressing is very helpful, and so a midwife must be chosen with lean hands and long fingers; and she will open the uterine opening, and when she sees the placenta, she has to tear it gently with her nails, and to put some suppositories with which to facilitate the birth without fear of **abortion**. Take suint, lily root, marjoram, calamint, two ounces of each one, and one ounce of terebinth, pound and mix them and wrap it up with wool so to make suppositories. And then she will be fumigated with cuckoopint, nutmeg; and then if all this has been done and still the birth is difficult, make her sneeze and be massaged forcefully. And if the woman is fat, she will kneel on her belly so that her knees touch her belly. And if the difficulty is caused by constipation of excrement, give her enemas, and if the reason is the stitching of the injury, there is no way other than to have the surgeon to cut it. And if the difficulty is caused by unnatural birth, bring the hand or leg back gently until the position is natural. And if the difficulty is caused by the death of the foetus, the woman should wash in water with pennyroyal, wormwood, marjoram, calamint, and should undergo the procedures mentioned in the above chapter on abortion. And if the reason for difficulty is diseases of the mother or clearly external reasons, these will be balanced by their opposites, as it has been mentioned above....

abortion: In premodern and early modern texts, the term was used both for intentional abortion of the fetus and unintentional miscarriages. You must read the text carefully to determine which is meant.

PART 10

Medicine and the Supernatural: Competitors or Partners? (ca. 1000–1400 CE)

In Parts 2 and 6 on ancient Greek and early medieval medicine, we can see examples of how supernatural and natural healing support each other or at least provide two different but acceptable paths of seeking a cure. This attitude persisted into the later Middle Ages, but there was occasional tension between miracles, magic, and medicine. The final documents in this collection (Documents 85–89) provide examples of religious or magical cures performed alongside of, or instead, of the more "natural" cures of healers and physicians. Also included are two documents (90 and 91) demonstrating the role of astrology in later medieval medicine.

As we can see in some sources (Documents 63, pp. 191–94, and 69, pp. 208–09), the city of Salerno in southern Italy was a famous center for healing and the education of physicians. By the twelfth century, "going to Salerno" could serve as a metaphor for hiring the services of a learned physician and buying expensive compound medicines. Modern historians still often call learned medieval medicine "Salernitan" even when it doesn't come from Salerno itself. It is thus telling that the miracle story in Document 85 presents a physician from Salerno (Hieronymus) and a saint (Trophimema), both of whom are called on to heal the girl Theodonanda. A similarly competitive but otherwise positive relationship between saint and physician can be seen in the saint's life of Milburga, or Mildburh (d. 715 CE), abbess of Wenlock Priory, a Benedictine monastery in England. She was venerated as a saint at her tomb, until it was destroyed by raiding Danes. Her bones were supposedly rediscovered in 1101, and several versions of her life and miracles were written after that, including the account in Document 86.

Until the twelfth century, most Christian saints became such by popular agreement, with the support of the local clergy. Such is the case with the early saints Cosmas and Damian, described above in Document 44, pp. 130–31. But in the later Middle Ages, the canonization of saints became an official process regulated by the Roman papacy. Saints had to be approved through an increasingly rigorous system of documentation and interviews. Many potential saints, especially women, did not pass the process. (They could still, however, be proclaimed as "venerable" or "beatified," and thus worthy of Christian admiration.) One such later medieval potential saint was Delphine, a noblewoman from Puimichel in southern France (1283–1360). The two statements in Document 87 come from her canonization proceedings, in which her neighbors claim to have been healed by her both before and after her death.

Many medieval people believed in the reality of magic, but it was often condemned as potentially demonic. Nonetheless, magical cures are relatively common in later medieval manuscripts (equally in Christian, Jewish, and Islamic cultures) and appear alongside the more acceptable forms of religious healing, like those in Documents 85–87. Certain forms of healing in the Middle Ages blurred the boundary between medicine, magic, and religion. There are many surviving examples of medieval healing charms, short stories or songs intended to be recited near or over the patient. They are little different from magical spells of healing from ancient cultures. Document 88 is a later medieval Hebrew treatment for a woman's infertility, copied in the margin of a later medieval Jewish rabbinical manuscript. Most of the document is a typical recipe, calling for the application of an herbal broth. However, the recipe becomes "medico-magical" through the addition of a German charm to be spoken to a pear tree, if the woman wants a male child, and the ritual incorporation of the mother's menstrual blood and another male child's umbilical cord. For comparison, Document 89 records three Christian medical charms from a twelfth-century manuscript. They explicitly invoke Christ and God, the Virgin Mary and the Christian saints and angels for curing paralysis, migraine, and wounds, rendering them more acceptable to the people of Christian medieval Europe.

The final two documents in this chapter reflect the common practice in the later medieval period of medical astrology, knowledge of which came primarily from the Arabic world in the twelfth and thirteenth centuries. While we might group together magic and astrology today as antiquated superstitions, most astrology was considered acceptable in the later Middle Ages so long as you attributed only influence, rather than direct causation, to the stars and planets. The stars had influence especially over water and other liquids, including blood and the other bodily humors, and thus astrology could be used to determine when was the best time to balance the humors through bloodletting or phlebotomy. While bloodletting had been practiced throughout the early and central Middle Ages in monasteries, the practice became widespread in the later medieval period and subjected to all of the latest medical theory. Bloodletting was one of the first lines of defense in balancing the humors, through the belief that the process removed corrupted or excess humors and allowed the body to create new, healthy blood.

John Arderne (1307–92) was a literate surgeon in England, roughly contemporary with Geoffrey Chaucer. Arderne described in his writings some surgical procedures that are still used to this day, most famously his treatment for anal *fistulae*, painful ulcers caused by sitting on horseback for long periods of time. But Arderne was also a healer of his time, which means he took seriously the influence of heavenly bodies, especially the twelve signs of the zodiac, on the human body. His instructions in Document 90 describe which zodiac sign "rules" over which body part. A surgeon should not cauterize or let blood from a body part when the moon is in that body part's zodiac sign, for the celestial forces will draw out more blood than the surgeon wants or further imbalance the patient's humors. Arderne refers to a drawing showing astrological signs in relation to parts of the body. This sort of image, known as a Zodiac Man or Bloodletting Man, was common in later medieval manuscripts and early printed books (Document 91), and became a standard part of the later medieval physician's toolkit.

DOCUMENT 85:

A Doctor and a Saint in Early Salerno[1]

> This miracle story presents a physician from Salerno (Hieronymus)
> and a saint (Trophimema), both of whom are called on to heal the girl
> Theodonanda. Since it is a miracle story, St. Trophimema obviously succeeds
> in healing, but the physician stills comes out looking as a wise, caring, and
> religious companion to the saint. This differs from some earlier miracle stories
> in which earthly physicians are made to look like criminals or quacks when
> set up against the healing power of saints. This miracle is placed in the ninth
> century, when we can date the prefect Pulchari, but it was recorded some time
> later, probably in the tenth or eleventh century.

೮

In the time of the most pious prefect Pulchari, a certain girl named
Theodonanda was given in marriage to a man named Mauro. Having con-
summated the marriage, because she was not yet nubile, she lay close to death
for a long time, each day she expected the wretched end to her torture. At
that time there was a powerful doctor, Hieronymus, providing good health
with the best medicines at Salerno. When her parents brought her to him,
in order that he might find some medicinal remedy for her, he rejected her,
saying, "Her illness is incurable, I will not be able to help her." They pleaded
with him to show her some pity and after several prayers, overcome, he asked,
"How long has this discharge troubled her?" They replied, "Four months.
Because of this, brought to desperation by her harsh misery, we came so
that, with the mercy of God, she might receive good health through you."

At those pleas the doctor, a servant of God, was overcome and began to
consult immense volumes of books on his art, to see if by chance he could
through reading recognize a cure for his illness: when he had read through
all his diseases, and could find nowhere which illness she was suffering
from, he said, "Go away from here brothers, because I cannot offer her any
medical help; know this, however; either she will be cured through the mercy
of God, or she will be punished through just judgement." Hearing these
words, they began to shed bitter tears, and bidding farewell they came to
Reginna so that, just as the doctor had said, they might mourn their dead.
And discussing their plight and coming to agreement they got up to take
her to the basilica of St Trophimema (it was not at all far from the same
church's enclosure). The girl was brought to the tomb of St Trophimema, a

---

1   Patricia Skinner, editor and translator, *Health and Medicine in Early Medieval Southern Italy* (Brill, 1997), 149, 151.

nun named Agatha took her and laid her womanishly in front of the altar,
praying, and then waited with her parents for three days for her to come
out. Such was the illness of her body that she waved her arms back and
forth ... laying down underneath just like a bird of prey calls with a long
flight in the air.

And when the girl was tired by these fatigues, her parents left her with
the nun, and she slept a little in front of the altar, and behold the girl went
out on tiptoe and headed for the river alone; for the hollow riverbed was
not yet hastened. And behold she saw the most beautiful girl of all, giving
her three blows on the back and saying, "Why have you dared to leave the
church, go back, and always fear me." When the agitated girl went back
and told the nun, she rejoiced ceaselessly, that St Trophimema had appeared
to her specially. Having sampled these benefits, the nun saw the pavement
sweating large quantities of oil, full of perfume, and prayed intently to God,
invoking the saint; she ordered the girl the undress and anointed her tiny
body with the holy oil, and immediately she was cured from her illness.

DOCUMENT 86:

The Life of St. Milburga: Physicians and Saints, Healing Together?[2]

> St. Milburga, or Mildburh (d. 715 CE), was the abbess of Wenlock Priory,
> a Benedictine monastery in England. She came to be known especially as
> a healing saint after her bones cured a woman who had already gone to a
> physician. Like the Italian physician above in Document 85, this English
> physician Ramelmus is presented in positive terms. He fails to heal this sick
> woman only because God wanted to use this one opportunity to reveal the
> goodness of Milburga.

ev

Now there lived in a village called Petelia a certain woman who for five
years had been languishing from the disease with which she was afflicted,
as was obvious to all from the pallor of her countenance and the abject state
of her body. And to this not a few of our brethren of good repute who had
frequently seen her before have most certainly testified to me. A member
of our congregation, Ramelmus by name, a most excellent brother, skilled in
the art of medicine, had often advised her and had supplied her with many
medicines; but these remedies which she had taken on his recommendation
had done her no good at all. For the Lord had deliberately reserved the
occasion of her cure in order to reveal his Saint. When she had drunk some
of the water in which the holy bones [of Milburga] had been washed she
immediately vomited a rather horrifying worm and from that moment was
completely restored to full health, so that to this very day both the bloom
of her complexion and the vigour of her whole body testify to how much
merit the Saint whose bones were discovered enjoys in the sight of God.
As for the worm, her husband, Oddo by name, brought it to the monastery
in a wooden box carved to the size of the worm. This wooden box I have
myself seen and handled. Many of the brethren came together to look at
the worm for it was quite unlike any reptile they had ever seen: it had twin
horns on its head, crawled on six feet and had another two horns also on its
tail. This was the beginning of the wonderful signs of the blessed Milburga,
by which her reputation began to spread far and wide. Meanwhile the sick
began to come in from distant towns and villages, some on horseback, some
indeed carried in litters from all over the country, so that the crowd of sick
could hardly be contained within that church and cemetery.

---

2   A.J.M. Edwards, "An Early Twelfth Century Account of the Translation of St. Milburga of Much
    Wenlock," *Transactions of the Shropshire Archaeological Society* 57:2 (1962–63), 134–51: 146.

Doctors and Miracles in the Canonization of Lady Delphine[3]

> The short documents below are depositions of witnesses in the canonization
> proceedings of Lady Delphine of Puimichel (1283–1360), in which her
> neighbors claim to have been healed by her both before and after her death.
> They reveal how later medieval people felt comfortable seeking professional
> physicians, self-help, and religious cures for the same ailment. Delphine was
> never approved as a saint, but these witness reports provide valuable evidence
> for the multiple forms of healing available in later medieval Europe.

ℰↄ

Delphine, While Alive, Heals Alacasia Mesellano

Again, Alacasia said that a good six years had passed, or thereabout, as it
seemed to her; she otherwise does not remember the month or day, since the
witness had a certain infirmity in the ring finger of her right hand, which is
commonly called *boblau*. It had a livid color and caused her great pain, and
sometimes she grew feverish from the pain of the said infirmity, and her
right hand swelled up, nor was she able to be freed [from the pain] using the
remedies which a doctor applied. And after she had the aforesaid infirmity
for eight days, she went one time to visit the aforesaid Lady Delphine. And
indeed the lady, seeing the finger of the witness herself wrapped up, because
the witness herself had applied a certain plaster, she asked what it was. And
the witness herself responded that she suffered pain in the aforesaid finger,
and she explained the aforesaid things to her Delphine. At the order of the
said Lady Delphine, she unwrapped the finger which was hurting. And then
the said Lady Delphine placed her hand on the hand of the said witness
and touched it and said to the witness herself that she should rebind the
said finger. And when Alacasia was in her house, she unwrapped the said
finger and found that it was totally cured.

3   Nicole Archambeau, "God Helps Those Who Help Themselves: Negotiating a Miracle in the
Fourteenth-Century Canonization of Delphine de Puimichel," *Anuarios de Estudios Medievales*
43:1 (2013), 7–25: 19, note 30, original translation by the editor of this volume; Nicole Archambeau,
"Miracle Mediators as Healing Practitioners: The Knowledge and Practice of Healing with Relics,"
Social History of Medicine 31:2 (2017), 209–30: note 80, original translation by the editor of this
volume.

Delphine's Hair, after Her Death, Heals Alasacia of Apt

Katherine also said that she saw Alasacia, whose last name she didn't know: she was living in the city of Apt and was rather deaf. And [there was] a doctor, hearing about the infirmity which Alasacia was suffering, as Alasacia had described it to the witness. And the witness herself had sent to her Alasacia some *oleo umbrino* for the purpose of curing the infirmity of her ears. Yet Alasacia herself did not use the oil, as she told the witness. But when she held some hairs of the said Lady Delphine (which, according to the witness, Katherine had given to Rixendis, the daughter of the said Alasacia, who petitioned her help on behalf of her mother, because she heard that the said witness had given some of the said hairs to the aforesaid **Ysoarda**), the said Alasacia was able to hear on that very day and on the following day the witness herself recognized, when she spoke to Alasacia, that Alasacia could hear her words.

oleo umbrino: Identity unknown, but the name suggests a specialized medical oil associated with the region of Umbria.

Ysoarda: Katherine's sister and wife of the local lord.

DOCUMENT 88:

Medieval Jewish Magical Medicine[4]

The following treatment for a woman's infertility was written primarily in Hebrew, but the italicized charm in the middle, addressed to a pear tree, is in German. It is recorded in the margin of a later medieval Jewish rabbinical manuscript. The first part of the description is not magical at all, and is quite similar to more mainstream gynecological treatments (see Documents 83 and 84 above), but the inclusion of a charm spoken to a pear tree makes this cure "medico-magical."

❧

A treatment for a barren woman. She should take [*here follows a list of ingredients and specified quantities*] and she should cook them with good strong wine in a large firm metal pot. And while the pot is still piping hot she should sit on the pot and do this three times a day for eight consecutive days so that the scent will penetrate her body through the uterus to warm the placenta. And then she should take her menstrual blood and place it in a vessel with some water. If she wishes to have a male child she should go to a pear tree and kneel before it as night turns to day and say to the tree: ***Birnbaum, ich klage Gott und dir dass mir ist genommen meine Frucht gif mir deine Frucht und nimm meine un-Frucht***. And she should pour her menstrual blood on the tree and repeat this for three consecutive mornings when night ends and day begins and then she should take a piece of the tree and cook it with water and take a male child's **navel** and crush it in the water and drink it.

Birnbaum ... un-Frucht: "Pear tree! I protest to God and to you for my fruit has been taken from me. Give me your fruit and take away my Infertility."

navel: The remains of the child's umbilical cord after birth.

4 Ephraim Shoham-Steiner, "'This should not be shown to a gentile': Medico-Magical Texts in Medieval Franco-German Jewish Rabbinic Manuscripts," in *Bodies of Knowledge: Cultural Interpretations of Illness and Medicine in Medieval Europe*, edited by Sally Crawford and Christina Lee (British Archaeological Reports, 2010), 53–59: 55.

DOCUMENT 89:
Medieval Christian Healing Charms[5]

Medieval healing charms were short stories or songs intended to be recited near or over the patient. They blur the boundary between medicine, magic, and religion, as Christian names and figures are invoked to ward off sickness. The name of the patient would be inserted where each charm reads ".N." for the Latin *nomen*, "name." These three charms come from a twelfth-century manuscript but variants of the "Three Good Brothers Charm" date back to the fifth century CE. In some versions of this last charm, the brothers are named and two are called Cosmas and Damian after the saintly physicians (see Document 44, pp. 130–31).

e

Angels against the Demons of Sickness

Nessia, Nagedo, Stechedo, Troppho, Crampho, Gigihte, and Paralisis: These curious names are personified Germanic terms for gout and rheumatism except for the Greco-Latin term *Paralisis*.

Three angels strolling on Mount Sinai encountered there **Nessia, Nagedo, Stechedo, Troppho, Crampho, Gigihte, and Paralisis**. The angels asked them: "Where are you bound?" "We are going," they replied, "to the servant of God .N. to torment his head, weaken his veins, suck his marrow, break his bones, and destroy his whole body." Then the angels said to them: "We adjure you Nagedo, Stechedo, Troppho, Crampho, Gigihte, and Paralisis by the Father, Son, and Holy Ghost, by the Blessed Virgin Mary, mother of God, by the apostles, martyrs, confessors, virgins, by all the saints and the elect of God, that you do not harm this servant of God .N. neither in the head, nor in the veins, nor in the marrow, nor in the bones, nor in any part of his body." Amen.

Saint Peter's Migraine

St. Peter sat on a marble block and put his hand to his head; he was miserable, exhausted by a toothache. Jesus appeared before him and said: "Why are you sad, Peter?" "Lord, the worm of migraine is eating up my teeth." Jesus said then: "I adjure you, O worm of migraine, by the Father, Son, and Holy Ghost, that you leave .N., the servant of God, and that you never again hurt him."

5   Edina Bozóky, "Mythic Mediation in Healing Incantations," in *Health, Disease and Healing in Medieval Culture*, edited by Sheila Campbell, Bert Hall, and David Klausner (St. Martin's Press, 1992), 82–92: 86–87.

The Three Good Brothers Charm

Three good brothers strolled on a road and the Lord Jesus Christ appeared before them and said: "Three good brothers, where are you going?" They replied to him: "Lord, we are going to the mountain to gather some herbs for wounds, bruises, and pains." And the Lord said: "Come with me and swear to me on the crucifix and on the milk of the Blessed Virgin not to reveal it in secret nor accept any reward for it. Go to the Mount of Olives and take some olive oil, soak some wool in it, and place it on the wound, saying thus: just as the soldier Longinus pierced the side of the Lord, and it neither bled long nor festered nor was painful nor swelled nor putrefied nor suffered inflammation, similarly let this wound, which I charm, neither bleed nor fester nor be painful nor swell nor putrefy nor suffer inflammation. In the name of the Father and of the Son and of the Holy Ghost." Amen.

DOCUMENT 90:

John Arderne, Astrological Instructions for the Surgeon[6]

> The English surgeon John Arderne (1307–92) became famous for his surgical treatment of anal fistulae, described in his book on this subject, *Fistula in Ano*. This work also describes many other conditions treated by later medieval surgeons and the procedures they used such as bloodletting, cautery, and cupping to balance or purge the humors. His instructions below describe which of the 12 signs of the astrological zodiac "rules" over which body part. A surgeon should not cauterize or let blood from a body part when the moon is in that body part's zodiac sign, for the celestial forces will draw out more blood than the surgeon wants or further imbalance the patient's humors.

∾

Ptolemy: A Greek mathematician and astronomer in the Roman Empire (ca. 100–170 CE), Ptolemy was best known in the Middle Ages for his book on astrology, the *Almagest*.

Pythagoras: Ancient Greek philosopher (ca. 570–495 BCE), revered in the Middle Ages as an early expert in mathematics, music, astronomy, and astrology.

Rhasis: Also Rhazes or Rasis, Latin spellings of the Islamicate physician and author al-Rāzī.

Haly: Short for Haly Abbas, a medieval European spelling and abbreviation of 'Ali ibn al-'Abbas al-Majusi, whose work was known best in Europe through the translations of Constantine the African (see Documents 62 and 66, pp. 188–90 and pp. 199–200).

The highest Astrologers, viz. [namely]: **Ptolemy, Pythagoras, Rhasis, Haly**, etc., aver that a surgeon ought not to cut or to cauterize any member of the human body nor to breathe a vein so long as the moon is in the house ruling that member. For the 12 signs of the Zodiac rule the twelve parts of the human body, as is clear from the aforementioned drawing, where Aries, which is a fiery sign moderately dry, governs the head with its contents. But when the moon is in Aries beware of operating upon the head or face and do not open one of the head veins. When the moon is in Taurus refrain from operating upon the neck or throat and do not bleed from a vein in these parts. When the moon is in Gemini beware of operating on the shoulders, arms or hands, and do not open a vein in these parts. When the moon is in Cancer refrain from operating upon the breasts or chest or stomach and from injuring the lungs, neither open an artery or a vein in their neighborhood. When the moon is in Leo take care not to injure the flanks or the ribs, and do not operate upon the back either by cutting or by cupping. When the moon is in Virgo take care not to operate upon the belly or the internal parts, and do not bleed from the veins supplying the womb in women. When the moon is in Libra refrain from operating upon the navel or upon the buttocks or upon the kidneys, and do not open the vein supplying the kidneys, nor apply a cup. When the moon is in Scorpio refrain from operating upon the testicles, the penis and the neck of the bladder; do not open the testicular vein and do not apply a cup. When the moon is in Sagittarius do not operate upon the thighs, do not remove spots or superfluous parts occurring in any part of the human body. When the

---

6   John Arderne, *Treatises of Fistula in Ano, Hemorrhoids, and Clysters*, edited by D'Arcy Power, Early English Text Society no. 139 (London, 1910), 17, 20.

moon is in Capricorn refrain from the knees and from injuring the veins and nerves in these parts. When the moon is in Aquarius do not operate upon the legs or upon their nerves from the knees to the bottom of the calves. When the moon is in Pisces do not operate upon the feet and do not open the vein in their extremities.

DOCUMENT 91:
Astrological Bloodletting Man[7]

This image, known as a Zodiac Man or Bloodletting Man, was common in later medieval manuscripts and early printed books. It shows the influence of each of the 12 zodiac signs on different parts of the body. The signs, like the humors and body parts, were defined by their elemental qualities. For example, Aries dominates the head, and is hot and dry, giving it a fiery and choleric aspect. This chart could be used to make a prognosis relating to the aspect of those body parts, and it was especially useful for determining whether bloodletting, cupping, or cautery should be performed.

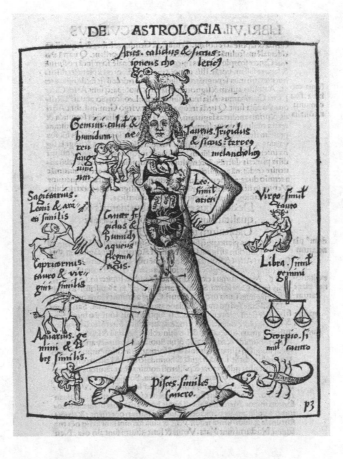

---

7   *De Astrologia*, from Gregor Reisch, *Margarita philosophica* (Freiburg, 1503). Image from the
    Wellcome Collection, wellcomecollection.org, licensed under the Creative Commons Attribution
    4.0 International License.

GLOSSARY AND INDEX OF KEY TERMS

Abortion: In premodern and early modern texts, the term was used both for intentional abortion of the fetus and unintentional miscarriages. You must read the text carefully to determine which is meant. See pp. 44, 52, 71, 124, 181, 241–42, 248.

Alvine: Relating to the belly or intestines. See pp. 40, 46–48.

Aposteme: A swelling or abscess filled with pus. See p. 213.

Asclepius/Asklepios: The Greco-Roman god of physicians. According to legend, he was the half-human son of Apollo and a mortal woman, taught the art of medicine by Chiron the Centaur. See Documents 13–18, pp. 52–61.

Basilic vein: One of the most important veins in premodern bloodletting, traveling on the surface of the inner arm from the shoulder down to the wrist. See p. 168.

Blood: In premodern Western medicine blood (Latin *sanguis*) could refer both to the pure humor of blood, representing the hot and moist qualities of the body, or the blood that flows through the veins, which is a composite of all four humors. Context is necessary to determine which *sanguis* the author intended.

Buboes: From the Greek *boubon*, "groin." Swellings of the lymph nodes, usually in the groin, armpits, or neck, are the best-known sign of plague in its bubonic form. See pp. 135–36, 204.

Calculus: a kidney or bladder stone. See p. 164.

Cancer: Ancient and medieval "cancer" (Latin *cancer*, Greek *karkinos*) included what we now know as cancer, but probably also a wide variety of tumors and lesions that "crept" along the skin like a crab (*cancer*) and were believed to be caused by black bile. See pp. 84–85.

Cautery: The application of burning hot irons to specific points on the body in order to modify the internal humors, such as through the removal or destruction of bad humors, or the creation of pus in the burn, which medieval physicians frequently saw as a beneficial sign. See pp. 205, 229, 262.

Choleric: Relating to yellow bile, *cholera*, and to anger, the emotion which was believed to be provoked by an excess of it. See pp. 154, 202, 262.

Coction/Concoction: The "cooking" of humors within the body, sometimes beneficial (as with the growth of children) and sometimes harmful (as with the corruption of humors leading to dangerous diseases). Coction is not to be confused with "decoction," a term for the preparation of herbal remedies by boiling or steeping the medicine. See pp. 41, 118, 175.

Collyria: Collyrium (singular), eye salves. See p. 178.

Complexion: One of the most important concepts in Hippocratic-Galenic medicine, complexion refers to the combination of qualities and humors in every person, plant, animal, or food. Only rarely does it have in medieval texts the modern sense of the tone and color of a person's skin. See pp. 30, 183, 188–94, 200.

Crisis: The turning point of a disease, either for better or worse. The term especially was used to refer to the point at which a patient's fever grew worst, broke, and led to recovery or death. See pp. 26, 39, 41, 47–48.

Cupping: The application of heated glasses to specific points on a patient's skin for the purpose of drawing out or shifting the internal humors. See also **Cautery** and **Phlebotomy**. See pp. 133, 137, 205, 260, 262.

Elephantiasis/*Elephantia*: Most likely leprosy, now known as Hansen's disease, but the term could apply to any number of conditions which cause extreme swelling of the limbs or very rough skin. See pp. 85, 202.

Erysipelas: Now a term for a specific bacterial skin infection, but in antiquity the term referred to a variety of inflamed skin rashes. See pp. 84, 173–74, 202.

Fumigation: The burning of a substance for medical purposes, to be inhaled or brought up into the uterus. See pp. 14, 78, 98–99, 241, 245, 248.

Galen: Claudius Galenus of Pergamon (ca. 130–ca. 210 CE) is generally considered the greatest physician of Western antiquity after Hippocrates. A Greek physician born in the Roman Empire, Galen practiced medicine in Rome itself, eventually serving as imperial physician to Marcus Aurelius. Galen saw himself as the direct heir of Hippocrates and wrote hundreds of medical and philosophical texts explaining Hippocratic texts and elaborating the humoral theory attributed to Hippocrates.

Hectic: A term used for intermittent, violent fevers, or for fevers arising from the corruption of the solid portions of the body. See p. 156.

Hippocrates: Hippocrates of Kos (ca. 460–370 BCE) was a Greek physician who practiced and taught medicine in Athens during the peak of classical Greece. A contemporary of Pericles and Socrates, Hippocrates is frequently considered the "father" of Western medicine for establishing a school of medical thought based on clinical observation and natural explanations for disease. Approximately 60 medical texts are attributed to his authorship although it is unclear if he actually wrote any of them.

Humoral medicine: Also known as humorism or humoralism, humoral medicine was the dominant medical theory in Europe and around the Mediterranean during classical antiquity and the Middle Ages, persisting well into the modern era until it was wholly supplanted by the germ theory of disease in the nineteenth century. Humoral theory argues that the human body contains four vital liquids, or "humors": blood, phlegm, yellow bile, and black bile. These humors must be kept in balance to preserve good health. According to humoral theory, disease is caused by the excess or imbalance of certain humors. The creation of this theory is attributed to Hippocrates and it was elaborated in the following centuries by his many admirers, especially Galen.

Hydromel: a mixture of honey and water commonly used in ancient and medieval medicine. See p. 79.

Hypochondrium/Hypochonder: The upper part of the abdomen, stretching over the lower ribs. The modern term hypochondria, referring to excessive or unfounded worrying about serious disease, was named after early modern patients who were convinced they suffered from an imbalance or corruption of humors in the hypochondrium. See pp. 47, 81.

Johannitius: The Latin rendering of the Arabic Hunayn ibn Ishaq, whose introduction to Galenic medicine, the *Isagoge*, served as the basis of learned medical education in Europe after it was translated into Latin by Constantine the African (see Document 52, p. 153). See pp. 149, 153–57.

Melancholy/Melancholic: Black bile (*melancholia*) and any disease engendered by that humor, which often produces sad feelings, hence the modern "melancholy." See pp. 83–85, 154, 191–94, 199–200, 202.

Methodism: An ancient medical school or "sect," best known from Galen's condemnation of their medical theories and practice. See pp. 69–70, 88, 94.

Oxymel: A common medical remedy, or base for other medicinal herbs, made of vinegar and honey. See pp. 169, 178.

Pessary: A medicated tampon made of cotton, cloth, or some other absorbent substance for insertion in the vagina or rectum. See pp. 52, 79, 99.

Phlebotomy: Cutting into a vein for the purpose of medical bloodletting, usually to balance the humors. Also called **Venesection**. The term is still used today for the process of giving blood.

Phlegm: One of the four primary humors of humoral medicine, representing the cold and moist qualities of the body. The mucus we now call phlegm is only one manifestation of this essential humor.

Phrenitis: An inflammation of the brain which was believed to produce "frenzy" (Latin *phrenesis*). See p. 98

Phthisis: Pulmonary tuberculosis. See pp. 44–45

Pituitous: Full of mucus or phlegm. See pp. 43–44.

Pleurisy/Pleuritic: Suffering from pleurisy, the painful collection of fluids or inflammation of the membranes around the lungs, called *pleurae*. See pp. 40, 43–44, 81–82.

Purgation/Purgative: A medicine or medical action designed to remove bad or excess humors from the body. These usually took the form of bloodletting or cupping, as well as drugs that caused vomiting, emetics for increased urination, or enemas. Women could also be prescribed emmenagogues, drugs that caused or increased menstruation.

Quartan: A fever which peaks and breaks every fourth day, measured inclusively (what we call every three days in modern counting). See pp. 31–32, 114, 156.

Quotidian: A fever that peaks and breaks once each day. See pp. 31–32, 156.

Refrigerants: Medications and medical procedures used by the Dogmatists to cool the body and slow the influx of excess fluid. See p. 68.

Regimen: A schedule of diet, rest, and physical activity prescribed by a physician, especially one trained in Hippocratic humoral theory. See Documents 22 and 63, pp. 40–41, 43, 46, 52, 69, 75, 157, 175, 177–78.

Sacred disease: Epilepsy was known as the "sacred disease" because many ancient people thought it was caused by a god or a spirit, an idea Hippocrates denies in his revolutionary work on epilepsy, *On the Sacred Disease*. See pp. 11, 39, 43.

Scrofula: Painful swelling of the lymph nodes, usually on the neck, and usually caused by tuberculosis. It was widespread in the Middle Ages and was known in Europe as the "King's Evil," because people believed that the touch of a king could cure it. See pp. 172, 221–22.

Semi-Tertian Fever/*Hemitritaeon*: A fever that peaks and breaks every day and a half (i.e., half of a **Tertian** fever). See pp. 100, 169.

Solution/Dissolution of continuity: A significant, negative, change or break in the composition of a part of the body. It usually means a wound or an ulcer. See pp. 226, 232.

Spirits: Intangible life forces which course through the body, not to be confused with the soul in the monotheist traditions. See pp. 153–54, 239.

Sternutatives: Substances that cause sneezing. See p. 94.

Strangury: Difficulty urinating or painful urination due to a blockage in the bladder. See p. 96.

Styptics: Like modern styptics, which are medicating agents designed to restrict blood flow and seal injured blood vessels, the styptic medicines of the Dogmatists were prescribed to constrict the flow of any fluid in the body. See p. 68.

Tertian: A fever that peaks and breaks every third day, measured inclusively (what we call every two days in modern counting). See pp. 31–32, 100, 114, 156.

Theriac: One of the most famous compound medicines of Antiquity and the Middle Ages, supposedly made of viper's flesh and numerous other exotic and expensive ingredients. It was believed to be a cure-all and every good apothecary, even up to the nineteenth century, carried a stock of theriac.

Venesection: Cutting into a vein for the purpose of medical bloodletting to balance the humors. Also called **Phlebotomy**.

FURTHER READING

This brief bibliography is restricted to books on ancient and medieval medicine written in English. Significant and important work on premodern medicine is being done in many other languages, as well as in journal articles and individual chapters within collections of essays, which are not included here.

Amundsen, Darrel W. *Medicine, Society, and Faith in the Ancient and Medieval Worlds.* Johns Hopkins UP, 1996.

Biller, Peter, and Joseph Ziegler, editors. *Religion and Medicine in the Middle Ages.* York Medieval Press, 2001.

Burnett, Charles, and Danielle Jacquart, editors. *Constantine the African and Ali ibn al-Abbas al-Majusi:* The Pantegni *and Related Texts.* Studies in Ancient Medicine, vol. 10. E.J. Brill, 1994.

Conrad, Lawrence I., Michael Neve, Vivian Nutton, Roy Porter, and Andrew Wear. *The Western Medical Tradition 800 BC to AD 1800.* Cambridge UP, 1995.

Corner, George Washington. *Anatomical Texts of the Earlier Middle Ages.* Washington, DC, 1927.

Demaitre, Luke. *Medieval Medicine: The Art of Healing, from Head to Toe.* Praeger, 2013.

Ferngren, Gary B. *Medicine and Religion: A Historical Introduction.* Johns Hopkins UP, 2014.

Ferngren, Gary B., and Ekaterina N. Lomperis. *Essential Readings in Medicine and Religion.* Johns Hopkins UP, 2017.

Finkel, Irving L., and Markham J. Geller, editors. *Disease in Babylonia.* Brill, 2006.

Flemming, Rebecca. *Medicine and the Making of Roman Women: Gender, Nature, and Authority from Celsus to Galen.* Oxford UP, 2001.

French, Roger. *Medicine before Science: The Business of Medicine from the Middle Ages to the Enlightenment.* Cambridge UP, 2003.

García-Ballester, Luis, Roger French, Jon Arrizabalaga, and Andrew Cunningham, editors. *Practical Medicine from Salerno to the Black Death.* Cambridge UP, 1994.

Geller, Markham J. *Ancient Babylonian Medicine: Theory and Practice.* Wiley-Blackwell, 2010.

Getz, Faye. *Medicine in the English Middle Ages.* Princeton UP, 1998.

Green, Monica H. *Making Women's Medicine Masculine: The Rise of Male Authority in Pre-Modern Gynaecology.* Oxford UP, 2008.

Grmek, Mirko D., editor. *Western Medical Thought from Antiquity to the Middle Ages,* coordinated by Bernardino Fantini, translated by Antony Shugaar. Harvard UP, 1998.

Hartnell, Jack. *Medieval Bodies: Life, Death and Art in the Middle Ages.* Wellcome Collection, 2018.

Horrox, Rosemary, editor. *The Black Death.* Manchester UP, 1994.

Jouanna, Jacques. *Hippocrates,* translated by M.B. DeBevoise. Johns Hopkins UP, 2001.

Kalof, Linda, editor. *A Cultural History of the Human Body in the Medieval Age*. Bloomsbury, 2010.

Kee, Howard Clark. *Medicine, Miracle and Magic in New Testament Times*. Cambridge UP, 1986.

King, Helen. *Hippocrates' Woman: Reading the Female Body in Ancient Greece*. Routledge, 1998.

King, Helen, editor. *Health in Antiquity*. Routledge, 2005.

Kirkham, Anne, and Cordelia Warr, editors. *Wounds in the Middle Ages*. Ashgate, 2014.

Krötzl, Christian, Katariina Mustakallio, and Jenni Kuuliala, editors. *Infirmity in Antiquity and the Middle Ages: Social and Cultural Approaches to Health, Weakness and Care*. Ashgate, 2015.

Longrigg, James. *Greek Rational Medicine: Philosophy and Medicine from Alcmaeon to the Alexandrians*. Routledge, 1993.

Longrigg, James. *Greek Medicine from the Heroic to the Hellenistic Age: A Source Book*. Routledge, 1998.

MacKinney, Loren. *Medical Illustrations in Medieval Manuscripts*. Publications of the Wellcome Historical Medical Library New Series Vol. 5, 1965.

Mattern, Susan P. *The Prince of Medicine: Galen in the Roman Empire*. Oxford UP, 2013.

McVaugh, Michael R. *Medicine before the Plague: Practitioners and Their Patients in the Crown of Aragon 1285–1345*. Cambridge UP, 1993.

McVaugh, Michael R. *The Rational Surgery of the Middle Ages*. SISMEL, 2006.

Mitchell, Piers D. *Medicine in the Crusades: Warfare, Wounds and the Medieval Surgeon*. Cambridge UP, 2004.

Nunn, John F. *Ancient Egyptian Medicine*. U of Oklahoma P, 1996.

Nutton, Vivian. *Ancient Medicine*. 2nd ed. Routledge, 2013.

Pormann, Peter, and Emilie Savage-Smith. *Medieval Islamic Medicine*. Georgetown UP, 2007.

Pouchelle, Marie-Christine. *The Body and Surgery in the Middle Ages*, translated by Rosemary Morris. Polity Press, 1990.

Scarborough, John. *Roman Medicine*. Thames and Hudson, 1969.

Scurlock, JoAnn. *Sourcebook for Ancient Mesopotamian Medicine*. SBL Press, 2014.

Shatzmiller, Joseph. *Jews, Medicine, and Medieval Society*. U of California P, 1994.

Wallis, Faith. *Medieval Medicine: A Reader*. U of Toronto P, 2010.

PERMISSIONS ACKNOWLEDGEMENTS

Bakhtiar, Laleh, adapter. From Volume 1 of *The Canon of Medicine (al-Qanun fi'l-tibb)*. Chicago: Kazi Publications, 1999. Reprinted with the permission of Kazi Publications.

Barkai, Ron. From "A Medieval Hebrew Treatise on Difficult Births," from "A Medieval Hebrew Treatise on Obstetrics," in *Medical History* 33 (1988): 96–119. Reprinted with the permission of Cambridge University Press via Copyright Clearance Center.

Behr, Charles Allison, translator. From *Aelius Aristides and the Sacred Tales*. Amsterdam: Adolf M. Hakkert, 1968. Reprinted with permission.

Black, Winston, editor and translator. From *Henry of Huntingdon, Anglicanus Ortus: A Verse Herbal of the Twelfth Century*. Pontifical Institute for Medieval Studies, Toronto. Reprinted with permission.

Black, Winston, translator. From "De atra bile," in *Claudii Galeni Opera Omnia*, Volume V, by Galen, edited by Karl Kühn. Leipzig, 1823, 119–22, 126–28, 130–31, 144.

Black, Winston, translator. From *Inventarium sive Chirurgia Magna*, Volume I, by Guy de Chauliac, edited by Michael R. McVaugh. Leiden: E.J. Brill, 1997.

Black, Winston, translator. From London, British Library, MS Sloane 1621, fol. 111r; and Bethesda (MD), National Library of Medicine, MS NLM E 8, fol. 10r, from Monica H. Green, "Making Motherhood in Medieval England: The Evidence from Medicine," in *Motherhood, Religion, and Society in Medieval Europe, 400–1400: Essays Presented to Henrietta Leyser*. Routledge, 2016, 179, fn 15.

Bos, Gerrit. From *Maimonides: Medical Aphorisms Treatises 1–5*. Brigham Young University, 2004. Reprinted with the permission of Brigham Young University.

Bos, Gerrit, translator. From Qustā ibn Lūqā on "The Little Dragon of Medina," in *Qusta Ibn Luqa's Medical Regime for the Pilgrims to Mecca. The Risala fi tadbir safar al-hajj*. Leiden: Brill, 1992. Reprinted with permission.

Bozóky, Edina. From "Mythic Mediation in Healing Incantations," in *Health, Disease and Healing in Medieval Culture*, edited by Sheila Campbell, Bert Hall, and David Klausner. Copyright © Centre for Medieval Studies, University of Toronto, 1992. Reprinted with the permission of SNCSC.

Brock, Arthur J., translator. From "On the Medical Sects," in *Greek Medicine: Being Extracts Illustrative of Medical Writers from Hippocrates to Galen*. London: J.M. Dent & Sons, 1929/Orion Publishing Group.

Bryan, Cyril P. From *Ancient Egyptian Medicine: The Papyrus Ebers*, translated from the German version. Chicago: Ares Publishers, 1974.

Corner, George W., translator. From "Anatomical Texts of the Early Middle Ages: A Study in the Transmission of Culture with a Revised Latin Text of Anatomia Cophonis and Translations of Four Texts." Washington, DC: *Carnegie Institution Publication 364* (1927): 51–53. Reprinted with permission.

Echols, Edward C., translator. From *History of the Roman Empire since the Death of Marcus Aurelius*, by Herodian of Antioch. Berkeley, 1961.

Edwards, A.J.M. From "An Early Twelfth Century Account of the Translation of St. Milburga of Much Wenlock," in *Transactions of the Shropshire Archaeological Society* 57, 2 (1962–63): 134–51. Reprinted with the permission of the Shropshire Archaeological and Historical Society.

Elgood, Cyril, translator. From "Tibb-ul-Nabi or Medicine of the Prophet," in *Osiris* 14 (1962): 33–192. Reprinted with the permission of the publisher, the University of Chicago. Copyright © 1962 The University of Chicago Press.

Grant, Mark. Excerpt from "Medical Compilations 4.11," in *Dieting for an Emperor: A Translation of Books 1 and 4 of Oribasius' Medical Compilations with an Introduction and Commentary.* Leiden: Brill, 1997, 2018. Reprinted with permission.

Green, Monica H., translator. From Chapter 8, Part 75 of *Medieval Italy: Texts in Translation,* edited by Katherine L. Jansen, Joanna Drell, and Frances Andrews. University of Pennsylvania Press, 2009. Reprinted with the permission of the University of Pennsylvania Press.

Hasan, Ahmad, translator. From Volume 3 of *Sunan Abu Dawud.* New Delhi: Kitab Bhavan, 2012.

Hitti, Philip K., translator. From *An Arab-Syrian Gentleman and Warrior in the Period of the Crusades: Memoirs of Usamah ibn-Munqidh (Kitab al-i'tibar), by Usamah ibn Munqidh.* Columbia University Press, 2000. Copyright © 1929, 1957 Columbia University Press; copyright © 1987 Princeton University Press; Copyright © 2000 Mrs. Viola H. Winder. Reprinted with the permission of the publisher.

Hooper, W.D. and H.B. Ash, translators. From *De Agricultura* by Cato. Loeb Classical Library, 1934.

Jones, W.H.S., translator. From *Hippocrates, Volume I (Airs, Waters, Places)* and *Volume IV (Aphorisms, Nature of Man).* London: William Heinemann, 1931.

Krueger, H.C. From *Avicenna's Poem on Medicine.* Springfield, IL: Charles C. Thomas, 1963.

Liuzza, R.M., translator and editor. From *Anglo-Saxon Prognostics: An Edition and Translation of Texts from London, British Library, MS Cotton Tiberius A.iii.* D.S. Brewer/Boydell & Brewer, 2011. Reprinted with the permission of Boydell & Brewer Ltd.

Meyerhof, Max. From "Thirty-Three Clinical Observations by Rhazes (circa 900 A.D.)," *Isis* 23, 2 (1935): 321–72. Reprinted with the permission of the publisher, the University of Chicago. Copyright © 1935 The History of Science Society.

Pines, Shlomo. From "The Oath of Asaph and Yoḥanan," from "The Oath of Asaph the Physician and Yoḥanan Ben Zabda—Its Relation to the Hippocratic Oath and the Doctrina Duarum Viarum of the Didachē," originally published in *Proceedings of the Israel Academy of Sciences and Humanities,* Vol. V, no. 9: 224–26. Jerusalem: The Israel Academy of Sciences and Humanities, 1975. Copyright © The Israel Academy of Sciences and Humanities. Reprinted by permission.

Riddle, John M. From *Dioscorides on Pharmacy and Medicine*. Copyright © 1985 by the University of Texas Press. Reprinted courtesy of the University of Texas Press. Excerpt from *Contraception and Abortion from the Ancient World to the Renaissance*. Cambridge, MA: Harvard University Press. Copyright © 1992 by the President and Fellows of Harvard College.

Shoham-Steiner, Ephraim. From "'This should not be shown to a gentile': Medico-magical Texts in Medieval Franco-German Jewish Rabbinic Manuscripts," in *Bodies of Knowledge: Cultural Interpretations of Illness and Medicine in Medieval Europe*, Studies in Early Medicine 1, edited by Sally Crawford and Christina Lee. Oxford: BAR Publishing, 2010, 53–59.

Skinner, Patricia, editor and translator. From *Health and Medicine in Early Medieval Southern Italy*. Leiden: Brill, 1997. Reprinted with permission.

Spencer, W.G., translator. From *De Medicina* by Celsus. Loeb Classical Library, 1938.

Spink, M.S. and G.L. Lewis, editors and translators. From *Albucasis on Surgery and Instruments: A Definitive Edition of the Arabic Text with English Translation and Commentary*. University of California Press, 1973. Copyright © 1972 by the Wellcome Institute of the History of Medicine. Reprinted with the permission of University of California Press.

Svarlien, Diane Arnson, translator. Excerpt from *Pythian 3, The Odes of Pindar*. Perseus Digital Library, http://www.perseus.tufts.edu/hopper/text?doc=Perseus:text:1999.01.0162:book=P.:poem=3. Reprinted with permission.

Temkin, Owsei, translator. From "Instructions for Midwives," in *Soranus' Gynecology*. Copyright © 1956, The Johns Hopkins University Press. Reprinted with the permission of Johns Hopkins University Press.

IMAGES

Cover Image: Wound man, Pseudo-Galen, Anathomia; WMS 290. Wellcome Collection. CC BY 4.0.

Page 195: Universitätsbibliothek Leipzig MS 1177, fol. 28 (fourteenth century). Credit: Wellcome Collection. CC BY 4.0.

From the Publisher

A name never says it all, but the word "Broadview" expresses a good deal
of the philosophy behind our company. We are open to a broad range of
academic approaches and political viewpoints. We pay attention to the
broad impact book publishing and book printing has in the wider world;
for some years now we have used 100% recycled paper for most titles.
Our publishing program is internationally oriented and broad-ranging.
Our individual titles often appeal to a broad readership too; many are
of interest as much to general readers as to academics and students.

Founded in 1985, Broadview remains a fully independent
company owned by its shareholders—not an imprint
or subsidiary of a larger multinational.

For the most accurate information on our books (including
information on pricing, editions, and formats) please
visit our website at www.broadviewpress.com. Our print
books and ebooks are available for sale on our site.

broadview press

www.broadviewpress.com

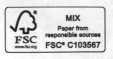 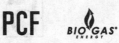